Short Essays on SEX

Short Essays on SEX

Dr. Vijai Rikh
Senior Sex Therapist and Consultant
Delhi

PEEPEE
PUBLISHERS and DISTRIBUTORS (P) LTD.

Published by
Pawaninder P. Vij
Peepee Publishers and Distributors (P) Ltd.
7/31, Ansari Road, Darya Ganj,
New Delhi - 110 002
Ph: 55195868, 9811156083
e-mail: peepee160@yahoo.co.in,
peepee160@rediffmail.com

First Edition: **2004**

ISBN 81-88867-07-1

Printed at
Lordson, C-5/19, Rana Pratap Bagh, Delhi - 110 007

To

My sister Chandra Bhushan

(Former Rajkumari of Tajpur)

and

My Brother-in-Law

Kulbhushan,

Who

rejoiced in my success

and

sympathized with me in my failures

I

sincerely

and affectionately

Dedicate

this book

Preface

'Sex' has been a tremendous force since time immemorial, but, surprisingly enough, we know very little about sex, about our sex organs.... How they work and how they are governed by a hormone known as 'Testosterone'. How we began our lives is all shrouded in mystery to millions of us.

We know more about our Motor Bike or Car, but know very little, what is happening two inches below our navel.

Though we are living in space age, but it looks we have left behind, our sex organs in stone age.

I shall feel duly rewarded, if by writing this book I am instrumental in bringing my readers somewhat closer to space age and enabling them to understand 'sex' in a much better way than before.

Before the advent of "Modern Sex Therapy" different sexual dysfunctions were taken as "fait accompli" but with new techniques, drugs and sex therapy the scenerio has dramatically changed and all sexual dysfunctions are now amenable to treatment and any body suffering from one or the other sexual disorder is sure to lead a complete, happier and contented sex life.

Dr. Rikh

Acknowledgements

I like to thank my wife Dr. (Mrs.) Kusum Rikh and my daughter Rita Rikh for their moral support, continued encouragement and inspiration, in writing this book, especially for editing and proof reading. I am sure without their assistance, it would not have been possible to complete this book.

And lastly special appreciation for my publisher Mr. Pawaninder P. Vij of Peepee Publishers & Distributors (P) Ltd. for putting up with my last minute alteration and additions in the manuscript and publishing this book within a very short span of time.

Dr. Rikh

Dear Reader,

This book 'Short Essays on Sex' is in your hand. Through these essays, I have endeavoured to bring before you the latest concepts and trends in 'sexology' by incorporationg some of the burning topics of the day. But, if inadverdently some other topics of interest have been left out, I would be pleased to include them in the next edition of the book, if intimated at the earliest, through publisher or direct to me by E-mail.

Dear reader, if you have any sexual problem, you can approach me on the addresses given below and I would be happy to be of some help to you in sorting them out.

With best wishes,

Dr. Rikh
C-2B/69A,
Janakpuri,
New Delhi - 110058

E-mail: drrikh@eth.net.
WWW.Indiansexologist.com

What the Great men say about

'Sex and Sexuality' ????

- Man can endure earthquake, dreadful disease, Epidemic, every form of spritual torment; but the most dreadful tragedy that can befall him is, and will remain, the tragedy of the bed room.

  ...***Leo Tolstoy***

- There is perhaps, no physial condition that is so humilating, so demoralizing, and so frustrating as Prematurev Ejaculation' and impotence.

  ...***Sexual Medicine today June '78***

- No civilized man is completely potent.

  ...***Sigmund Freud***

- Use it or lose it.

  ...***James Fries***

- On the ashes of yesterday, let us plant the oaks of tomorrow.

  ...***Anon***

- He who cannot embrace a women with dominant virility will be neither respected by her nor loved.

  ...***Michelet***

Contents

Chapter-1

The Penis and it's size

In the estimation of many men, their penis is the most precious organ they possess. So long as the heart goes on beating regularly, one takes it for granted; only if the lungs are not working properly, do we give them a thought; and so we regard liver and spleen, kidneys and bladder, eyes, ears and throat and the circulation of our blood.

The penis, however, we cannot forget. It forces its attention on us frequently; and it is the symbol of our self-esteem, for we base our self-esteem, not on what we achieve by brains or hands, but upon the quality of our manhood.

It stands to reason, therefore, that if anything goes wrong with our penis, which threatens to prevent it from expressing our manhood, as we believe it should be expressed, we fly to its aid and assistance more quickly than we rush to the doctor for his assistance with a wounded arm or leg.

I have before me as I write this, a letter from a man who says, 'my penis when erect is only 8 inches long. I feel I must make it longer. Please can you tell me how?' and I have in my files letters from men whose erect penises measure 3 ½ to 4 inches who are clearly genuinely concerned, and underlying their concern one can discern not only fear or inadequate performance or of not satisfying their partner, but fear of being laughed at by members of their own sex, and their partners.

The concern about penis-size is almost as old as man. For hundreds of centuries penile length and bulk has been the yardstick whereby man has measured his manhood and had his manhood assessed by his fellows. The erotic art of ancient civilizations has always depicted men with phenomenally large penises, and this convention has been carried down to the present day, not only in art of this nature, but in pornographic literature. Men who are concerned with the size of their penises, then, are in a long line of men of all times and races.

In this century concern about penis size has assumed a new characteristic. Men are now more concerned with being successful lovers than with producing strong and healthy and numerous children. Pride in their sexual adequacy – a very justifiable pride – is still centered on the penis, and it seems that psychologically men who consider themselves under endowed are particularly vulnerable.

Though every penis conforms to a basic shape, its length and girth vary from individual to individual as much as noses, ears, hands, and feet vary. There have, however, been numerous surveys of penile length and girth which have purported to be able to establish an average size; and according to these surveys, which tally remarkably closely, the average-sized penis among white men when fully erect measures a fraction above 6 inches in length and about 4 ¼ inches in circumference. There are quite a number of 7-inch penises, but 8-inches-and above are rare, while the few 9-inches that exist ought to be museum exhibits. There are about as many 4 ½ to 5-inch penises as there 7-inch plus penises, while below 4 inches are as rare as 8-inch-and-above.

The American researchers Dr. William H. Masters and Mrs. Virginia E. Johnson, however, have recently made an important discovery. After measuring several hundred penises of all lengths, they have reported that it would seem that *the longer the limp penis the less its length increases proportionately in erection than the smaller penis,* e.g. 3 ½ inches when relaxed may when erect go to 5 ½ or 6 inches, while the man with the 5- or 6-inch limp penis may have an erect penis of 6 ½ to 7 inches. They report one case of a 3-½ inch limp penis, which in erection increased by 120 per cent of 7 ½ inches; and another of 4 ½ inches with an erect length of 7 inches.

The great point of this discovery is that it confirms what sexologists have been insisting for a long time – that the man with the small limp penis, which is what his fellows may see, should not let it become a psychological block; and it emphasizes that it is the length of the erect penis which counts.

But how far it counts is another matter, too. Let me state here and now and categorically that the only men who have just cause for complaint are those whose erect penis is 3 inches or less. Anything above this measurement is fully capable of giving any woman complete satisfaction.

Let us examine the facts. The average length of the vagina when the woman is not roused is 3 ½ inches. Masters and Johnson's researches have revealed that when she is sexually roused, the vagina automatically lengthens by about an inch, or perhaps a little more. This means that the 4 ½ -inch penis completely fills the vaginal barrel. The extent to which the average 3-½ -inch vagina can be stretched without the woman being more than ordinarily aware of it is 6 to 6 ½ inches, which represents almost the limit of possible male penetration, the vaginal tissues then being at full stretch. It is only when the vagina is stretched to 7 ½ to 8 inches that the woman experience any sensations of stretching, and she may not do so even then.

The only part of the vaginal barrel, which is sensitive, is the first third of its length, from the vagina entrance: what Masters and Johnson call the orgasmic platform. It is, therefore, her experience of the penis in this first third, which will make any impression on her. Supposing when she is roused her vagina automatically lengthens to, say, 6 inches, which is far in excess of the average. Her orgasmic platform even then is 2 inches long, and a penis of only 3 ½ inches will make contact with the vital area, with some to spare.

Now, it is a fact that as climax approaches there is often a psychological desire on the part of both partners for deeper penetration. This desire is psychologically fulfilled by the partners straining their pubic areas against one another, which gives the impression to both of deep penetration, whether there is actual stretching beyond the normal limit of the vaginal tissue by a 7-inch penis or not. The man with the average 6-inch penis completely satisfies his partner's penetration desire; the man with the 7-inch penis stretches the vaginal tissue to just that degree that is tolerable for the woman; the 8-inch penis goes beyond the tolerance limit, and sets up sensations which very few, if any, women can accept.

This clearly demonstrates that 7 inches is the maximum length, which can give a woman pleasure. Anything beyond 7 ½ inches, i.e. 8 or 9 inches, gives her pain, and if the few 8-inch men will be absolutely honest, they will confess that they do not at any time use the full length of their penis.

In other words, the average 6-inch penis gives really deep penetration, the 7-inch borders on the excessive, while anything above that is useless and might just as well not be there. On the other hand, even the 3 ½ inch penis makes contact with more than the vital first third of the vaginal barrel in which the woman is conscious of its presence, and can respond to the psychological urge for deeper penetration by the firm pressure of the two pubic areas against one another.

Penile length, therefore, has No significance whatsoever either in performance or capacity for satisfying the woman. It has significance only for those men who have become obsessed with it.

Chapter-2

Premature Ejaculation

One man out of every eight, perhaps, suffers from the uncontrollable premature ejaculation of semen. It is probably the most common disturbance of male potency and one of the greatest causes of unhappiness in marriage. If it persists untreated over a long period of time, it can lead to impotence.

There are two forms of this condition, which is known medically by the Latin term, *ejaculatio praecox'*. The involuntary ejaculation of semen immediately upon introduction of the penis into the vagina, or so soon afterward that the female has no opportunity to reach orgasm, is known as *ejaculatio post portas*.

A more serious form is *ejaculatio ante portas,* in which ejaculation occurs before the penis is introduced into the vagina. There may be an ejaculation without any erection, when kissing the sexual partner, perhaps, or merely from being close to her.

The semen may flow like urine from a relaxed organ. Or it may be expelled while the penis is in a semi-erect state.

A prolonged period of premature ejaculation is a serious matter. The condition is often accompanied by periods of temporary impotence. Untreated, it may lead to very real impotence.

The man, who is unable to delay ejaculation and thus complete a sexual union satisfying to his wife and to him, soon begins to feel inadequate. Each failure leads to the expectation of another failure. This creates a state of tension, which make successful intercourse unlikely.

Because the male is so sensitive about his potency, many men do not seek medical help for premature ejaculation. Often, a sexually frustrated wife complaining of vague "nervous" ailment brings the situation to the attention of the family physician. Or an unhappy woman seeking to save her marriage—or to dissolve it-blurts out her distress to a marriage counsellor or an attorney.

The majority of cases of premature ejaculation are caused by a hypersensitivity of the male sexual mechanism. Ejaculation is a reflex, the response to intense sexual stimulation. When the male's sexual mechanism is supersensitive, this reflex mechanism is unusually rapid; the body's response is swifter than the man wants it to be.

The hypersensitivity may be a physical one; the head of the penis may be so extremely sensitive that orgasm occurs almost as soon as the organ touches the female genitals.

It may be an emotional one; both the man who is intensely passionate and the man who harbors some mild anxiety about sex may be unable to tolerate intense sexual excitement, except briefly.

For many years, physicians have been searching for an effective treatment for premature ejaculation. Various methods have been tried, with varying degrees of success.

Anesthetic ointments have been used. Applied to the glans penis before intercourse, they make that organ less sensitive and able to withstand longer contact with the vagina.

Tranquilizers have been useful in some cases, hypnosis in others, and men have been taught – or have taught themselves—all kinds of tricks to distract them from the sexual act and thus, perhaps, delay orgasm.

One patient of mine found doing complicated mathematical problems in his head a good delaying tactic. Another would silently recite the alphabet backwards.

But these methods were not completely successful, or they were successful with some men and not with others, or they worked only temporarily.

Now, however, physicians have found a new approach to these major sexual problems, an approach that gives vast promise of cure.

This treatment, too, is based on the theory of desensitization. But it does not require use of a pharmaceutical or psychological desensitizing technique at the time of every intercourse.

Instead, it aims at permanently curing premature ejaculation by retraining the man's pattern of sexual response so that a greater—and more usual—amount of sexual stimulation is needed to trigger the ejaculatory reflex.

There are two methods using this re-training technique. Both are simple; they sound almost surprisingly simple. Both can be used either by husband or wife who are willing to cooperate to overcome the problem. And-perhaps best news of all to those whose marriages are made miserable by the problem of premature ejaculation—improvement is rapid.

The first method takes what we may call the active approach. It was developed by Dr.James H. Semans of Duke University School of Medicine.

This method requires the wife to stimulate the male organ manually until the husband becomes aware of the sensation that immediately precedes ejaculation. He then signals his wife, who immediately ceases the stimulation. When the sensation has disappeared, the wife again resumes the stimulation; again, her husband has her halt when he feels the sensation, which tells him ejaculation is about to occur.

Repeating this procedure establishes a pattern of sexual response in which intense stimulation is tolerated and ejaculation is delayed. Soon, the man finds himself able to postpone ejaculation almost indefinitely.

Because ejaculation occurs more quickly when the male organ is wet than when it is dry, Dr. Semans advises the man to lubricate his organ with a bland cream when repeating the desensitizing technique.

This insures that ejaculation won't occur prematurely when the male organ is introduced to the moist surface of the vagina during normal coitus.

The second, or *passive approach* was developed by Dr. Joseph Wolpe, a practicing psychiatrist and a member of the medical faculty at the University of Virginia.

Dr. Wolpe found that impotence and premature ejaculation were often caused by anxiety or fear of the sexual situation. This anxiety is very easily stimulated. The man who is exceptionally fearful that he will not be able to perform intercourse successfully, for instance, may be so sensitive to any sexual situation that merely kissing the woman he desires arouses this fear and triggers the ejaculatory reflex.

He also found that desensitizing the man to these situations so that they were no longer very disturbing, enabled him to tolerate them without ejaculating prematurely.

Unlike the Semans' technique, Dr. Wolpe' method does not require the wife to stimulate her husband actively. As a matter of fact, it insists that nothing at all be done to increase his sexual excitation and that no sexual demands be made of him.

The recommended procedure is for the husband and wife to engage in sexual closeness without either expecting intercourse. In bed, they are to indulge in only as much sexual activity as the man can tolerate without anxiety. He is to do only as much as he really feels like doing, and no more.

Because there is no set goal he must reach, no level of sexual performance he must attain, the anxiety he feels about sexual situations is lessened.

As he becomes more relaxed he is able to indulge in more intense sexual embraces without becoming anxious. He is able to tolerate a greater amount of stimulation without ejaculation. His sexual mechanism has been re-trained so that it responds in the marital union with a greater degree of excitation and much less anxiety.

Both the active and passive approaches to this method appear to work exceedingly well; cures have been reported after a few weeks, at most a few months. In one case treated by Dr. Semans, a man who had suffered from premature ejaculation during all five years of his marriage was given instructions in the use of the technique. After five weeks, he and his wife reported that marital relations were mutually satisfying.

In case reported by Dr. Wolpe, a man who was troubled by premature ejaculation, which occurred before intromission, had been unwilling even to attempt intercourse for four years.

After repeated exposures to the sexual situation under the

conditions prescribed by the technique, he became less worried about his inability to perform. Eight months later, he and his wife were enjoying normal sexual relations.

Both techniques require the complete cooperation of the wife, and her utmost patience. Neither will work unless she is willing to help, unless she remains affectionate and encourageing and refrains from criticizing or making sexual demands.

In the method advocated by Dr. Semans, the procedure is to interview the husband and wife separately, to explain the technique and give instruction in its use, and then to see both together to make certain the instructions have been completely understood. After a few weeks, the man and his wife are interviewed again so that progress can be evaluated.

Dr. Wolpe recommends that the husband explain the situation to his wife, quoting the doctor if necessary.

With the use of either technique, premature ejaculation may accidentally occur, of course. The couple is advised to expect this. Because they no longer regard it as a sign of failure, it does not create tension or arouse the man's feelings of inferiority.

If premature ejaculation accidentally occurs during the procedure, DR. Semans advises that all further efforts be delayed, except that the husband is to manually stimulate his wife's clitoris until she reaches completion. He considers that helping the wife achieve sexual relief is something the husband must do if he is to get her continued cooperation. With the Wolpe method, the man is not required to perform any lovemaking except that which he freely desires.

One further word: The Semans and Wolpe approaches to the treatment of premature ejaculation work only in certain cases. Sometimes, premature ejaculation is a sign that all is not well with the patient's general health, and attention to the man's general well being solves the problem. Sometimes, it is a symptom of a deep-seated fear or hatred of women. In such cases, psychiatric treatment is necessary.

Every man suffers from premature ejaculation at one time or another in his sexual life when he is worried, or fatigued.

There is even a form called "honeymoon impotence" which occurs on the wedding trip, when both husband and wife are tired, tense and apprehensive.

If premature ejaculation occurs infrequently, and if there are long periods of satisfying sexual relations between the occasions on which it does occur, there is nothing to worry about.

But whenever it causes concern or marital discord, or is prolonged, medical advice should be sought. Only a Sexologist can determine which method of treatment is best for the individual case.

Chapter-3

Masturbation

About four decades ago, masturbation was considered as harbinger of sexual debility, premature ejaculation and importence. But after Kinsey report in 1953, the whole concept seems to be changed and it is not considered as such.

Now-a-days there are two schools of thought. One the old one is totally against masturbation. And the new school considers masturation as biological necessity and sees no harm in it, even if practiced daily.

New School

Usually boys become sexually mature at about 15 when their internal sex organs (glands) begin to produce their secretions (semen) needed for intercourse, and thus they are physiologically prepared for intercourse with females. Now their sexual instinct also starts working energetically and the boys feel an inner urge for intercourse. In the natural form of sex life among the savages the boys of 15 or older have intercourse regularly with different girls and in lower civilized society also when boys of 15 to 18 are married they have intercourse daily, and scientific research (Kinsey report, to be mentioned soon) has shown that human males are sexually most active and energetic (most powerful) at about the age of 16 to 17 so that at this age they can have intercourse more frequently than at any other age. But the modern young men receiving higher education are in schools and colleges at this age and so their marriage is delayed up to 25 or so, and the society prevents them from having intercourse before marriage. When the healthy sexual urge overpowers the minds of these youths they automatically think of and imagine intercourse with the females (working of the sexual instinct), the penis becomes erect, and then the boys further stimulate it by hand. Such handling of the penis further arouses them sexually and makes the picture of sexual intercourse clearer in their mind and after some movements of the hand holding the penis they get their orgasm and discharge semen resulting in the relief of their overpowering sexual urge (sexual relief). This practice is called *masturbation or self-relief;* and as we shall see later on, it is practiced by over 95% school and college-youths. Some of them practice it in a little different forms-by pressing the penis between the thighs or by rubbing or stroking it on the bed, etc.

The mind of the most young men is found infected with the pathogenic misbelief that masturbation injures or weakens the penis and/or makes the semen thin. The new school tries to destroy this misbelief and to show that masturbation is harmless.

Biologists and sex specialists are agreed that masturbation in such cases, practiced as a substitute for intercourse (a sort of imitation intercourse or imaginary intercourse), is quite harmless and almost inevitable, and that it relieves the sexual tension of the youths (which they periodically feel in absence of intercourse) and eases their minds so that they are able to pay better attention to their studies. Without such occasional relief their mind becomes tense and uneasy and keeps on thinking and Imagining of sexual affairs, and thus their studies and even sleep may be disturbed by sexual thoughts and persistent erections.

But in the lower class literature on sex, health and 'Brahmacharya' based on primitive child-like way of thought it is said that this practice of masturbation ruins the health of the body and mind, and boys in schools and colleges usually read such sort of literature, and usually they read it after they have begun masturbation. In this literature, as Brahmacharya is praised to the skies, masturbation is described as a devilish, bad and harmful practice often in a very frightening and terrifying way; and reading it, simple-minded ignorant boys are frightened and terrified that their health would now go to ruin as an after-effect of masturbation. Later on as a result of this foolish belief and fear continued for months and years they get various sorts of sexual troubles as well as bodily and mental troubles, and as time goes on this foolish belief and fear becomes so deep-rooted that it becomes difficult to remove it. This long continued anxiety and fear of losing health and of becoming impotent in many cases seriously disturbs the minds of these ignorant boys so that they become rather insane or crazy in this matter and go on saying foolishly, "The horrible practice of masturbation has ruined me completely." But this belief and fear acquired by reading that foolish literature on Brahmacharya is absolutely wrong and *must be removed,* for this itself is the cause of all sexual troubles. It is a very harmful pathogenic misbelief.

It is not only one who says so, all modern scientific authorities on this subject (biologists, psychologists, sexologists, sex specialist doctors etc.) are agreed that masturbation is quite harmless and that it is the fear and anxiety (worry) aroused by that foolish literature on Brahmacharya etc. that does the harm (which ignorant boys believe to be done by masturbation). So far you have been living in the darkness of the underworld of superstition and blind-faith, reading different books of this lower class; the following opinions will show you that there is a higher world of science and real knowledge (which you should now enter if you want health and happiness), they would lead you from darkness to light Perhaps you have been praying: -From darkness lead me to light, here is the answer to your prayer. I release a flood of light of scientific information to enable you to see your sexual problems clearly.

Kinsey Report. In the U.S.A. there is an institution under the Indiana University, named the *Sex Research institute,* which studies and investigates the sexual matters scientifically. Among its staff of several scientists Prof. A.C. Kinsey was the leading figure; he was a great biologist having outstanding intellectual ability and a vast general scientific knowledge, and was the professor of animal biology in that university. For about nine years these scientists studied the sex lives of 12000 persons (5300 males) of all ages and different parts of the U.S.A. by confidential and very tactful questioning (often examining the sex organs personally). In each case history 521 items were explored which cover all aspects of the sex life—sexual activities of young children, masturbation, night discharges, homosexual practices, intercourse with friends and companions of the opposite sex, with prostitutes, with animals; and all these things at what age began, how done and how frequently etc. etc. They have reported their findings in the form of two large books named *Sexual behaviour in The Human Female.* (Henceforth for the sake of brevity I shall refer to these books as Kinsey report, or Kinsey research.) No doubt they are the best books on the sexual matters, and would remain so for many years. Such outstanding books on sex come out hardly once in a decade. Those who are really interested in knowing facts about the sex life must read these books.

Dr. Edwin Hirsch, M.D., of the U.S.A., author of several books on sex, writes on publication of the first of these books, "During the past year a momentous change has been brought about in the average individual's attitude towards sexual relations. A new and penetrating light has been thrown on this subject by a very excellent piece of investigational study known as *Sexual behaviour in the human Male* by Dr. Kinsey. Never before has any book on sex received so much acclaim... Immediately the book became a best seller. In professional as well as in lay circles the book created a furor. Over every tea-and bridge-table the subject of conversation was the Kinsey report. The Kinsey report helps bring to a halt the destructive forces of sexual fear (that masturbation has made you impotent and weak)."

Here we are concerned with this book on the male only; besides other information it contains 162 revealing tables and 173 figures (graphs) showing how men of different ages, education and social status satisfy their sex desire, in what sort of activities they indulge, what percentage of them does so and how .frequently etc. etc. On masturbation this book says:

"About 92% of the total population is involved in masturbation which leads to orgasm. More individuals (96%) of the college level and 95% of the high school level are included and only 89% of those who never go up to high schools." It says that these youths of lower society satisfy their sex desire more by intercourse, which is not so easily available in the higher educated society. The remaining 5% youths of colleges and schools do not masturbate because they do not have enough sexual desire (are rather weaklings) or have intercourse etc. More educated boys masturbate, for it requires imagination to get pleasure in this way, and the dull minded uneducated boys do not have so much imagination. Some dull minded and uneducated boys cannot bring about discharge by masturbation.

Of course, like other scientific authorities, these scientists of the Sex Research Institute consider masturbation quite harmless, and say that parents need not warn their boys against it and go on—"In as much as nearly all boys arrive at masturbation sooner or later, it may be asked why one should worry over pre-adolescent or even infantile masturbation... If it is a question of physical outcome (harm) the issue is for the biologist, and it should be made clear that there is no evidence in the thousands of histories now at hand that the boy who begins masturbation at an early age suffers any more harm than the boy who delays the beginning of this experience until some time in adolescence or later. And most scientists and clinicians are now agreed that masturbation does no harm at any age." They mean that all healthy energetic boys practice masturbation, some begin it at an early age (of 8 or 9) and others later on at 16 or after that and it is rather necessary when sexual intercourse is not available, for no one can and no one should suppress his sexual impulse completely.

"There are a few males who masturbate only once or twice in their lives; there are others who have frequencies that may average seven to fourteen or twenty or more per week for long periods of years...Some males may masturbate several thousand times as often as some others in the population. The statement about the lack of harmful outcome still applies to these most active cases. (They mean that even in those who practice twenty or more times week masturbation causes no harm.) In the present records the highest rating males were masturbating with average frequencies of 23 per week in early adolescence. These maximum average frequencies drop to 15 per week by twenty years age, to 6 per week by fifty years of age, and to once in two weeks at sixty years of age... For the active population, average frequencies of masturbation are nearly two per week, but a good number (17%) of boys at that age may average four to seven times a week or oftener. A much larger number of boys reach these higher frequencies on occasions even though they do not regularly average such rates.

"In the present study we have examined the histories of

5300 males of which 5100 record experience in masturbation. It would be difficult to show that masturbatory activities have done any measurable damage to any of the individuals...

"The average adolescent boy is quite capable of three or four ejaculations per week, and there are boys who are capable of seven to fourteen or more per week... Like many other physiologic functions, erotic response depends on a remarkably foolproof mechanism. When one reaches the limit of physiologic endurance he no longer responds erotically. He is no longer capable of erection and finds little incentive to force the situation..." They mean that no one can indulge in masturbation excessively so as to injure his sex organs or general health, just as no one can eat too much to injure his stomach.

Age and Sexual Capacity. They conclude that males are sexually most active at about the age of fifteen and the boys of this age can have intercourse more frequently than their fathers aged about 35 or 40. The belief that one is sexually most energetic in the middle twenties is found wrong. One attains his maximum sexual capacity before he is 18 and then it slowly begins to decline. Intercourse, masturbation and/or night discharges occur most frequently between the age of 14 and 18, and those boys who mature early (at 8 to 11 years) are sexually most capable and have intercourse, masturbation etc. More frequently and up to a more advanced age than those who mature late (at 15 years of age or later).

They say: "Not only do these early developing boys have four years' head start, and not only do they have higher rates of activity in those initial years, but they continue to have higher rates throughout the subsequent period. In the fifteen years that lie between the ages of 16 and 30, the younger developing boys have about half again as much outlet (intercourse, masturbation etc.) as the later developing boys. There is still a discernible difference in the age group 31 to 35, which is 20 to 25 years after the time of onset of adolescence! Considering the multiplicity of other factors that may modify the frequencies of sexual activities, it is surprising to find such a long-time correlation with the age of onset of adolescence. In spite of their early start, and in spite of their much higher expenditure of energy in sexual activity, these early maturing males remain more active than those who were delayed in adolescence... There is some reason for thinking that these early adolescent males are more alert, energetic, vivacious, spontaneous, and physically active, socially extrovert and/or aggressive individuals in population. Scientists in their study of geniuses found that the individuals with the highest IQ's (most intelligent) were those who became adolescent first...

You will see that it all goes to disprove the doctrine of Brahmacharya, which says that only those are mentally, and physically well developed who do not discharge their semen at least up to the age of 25, and who completely suppress the sex desire. You should know that these scientists are here giving the actual statistics, the facts discovered by them while making an objective study of the lives of 5300 people. Of course these facts are in harmony with the principles of biology.

Even ignorant boy misguided by the religious view of sex life believes that only he or a few other bad boys practice masturbation, and so every such ignorant boy feels guilty and ashamed for his practice of masturbation. Facts found by this scientific investigation should remove the unnecessary feelings of guilt, shame and fear (of harm to health) of these boys. And besides these scientists, there have been others in Europe, America and India who have investigated the facts about masturbation; they also report similar percentages (Havelock Ellis gives a summary of these reports in his book). Meirowsky (inquiry among doctors) reports that 90.7 per cent practice masturbation, Marcuse (Munich) reports 93.3 per cent, Deutsch (Budapest): 96.7 per cent, Prof. Duck (a British school doctor): 90—95 per cent, Dr. Hirschfeld (Berlin) 96 per cent, Brockmann who inquired among 232 Theological (religious) students: 99.3 per cent, Robie: 99 per cent, Dr. Stekel says every man masturbates. The Indian sexologist, Dr. A.P. Pillai, has similar opinion about masturbation among the Indian youths (96 per cent).

Considering all these facts it would be foolish if you still think that you have done something bad, shameful or harmful in practicing masturbation. Again, according to followers of new school *almost all healthy boys practice masturbation if they cannot have intercourse, and it is quite harmless.* To impress this fact on your mind and to remove your fear (that the masturbation you have practiced is going to harm your health) they quote the opinions of many other good sex specialist doctors. The opinions of these best doctors on the subject should remove wrong belief and fear that masturbation has harmful effects. *Unless this wrong belief and fear is removed one's sexual troubles cannot be cured* (for they are being causes by this wrong belief and fear).

Doctors' Opinions that masturbation is Harmless:

Dr. A.P. Pillai, M.B.B.S., O.B.E., author of several books on sex and sexual disorders, editor of the *International Journal of Sexology,* practicing as a sex-specialist for about 25 years, writes: "Well-meaning friends, both medical and non-medical, whose opinions I value, have leveled criticisms about my previous books. Some of these are that I treat most sex disorders as problems that need education rather than diseases that need treatment, that I am far too ultra-modern in my unequivocal teaching that auto-erotic practices (masturbation) lead to no permanent injury to the body, mind or sexual system and so on. I maintain that my attitude is right and my accumulating experience makes me still further convinced that it is so (that masturbation causes no harm).

"As regards auto-erotic practices (masturbation) and potency, I need only repeat what I have been maintaining all these years, and that is, I have not come across a single case where a man's impotence or a woman's frigidity can be attributed directly to autoeroticism. On the other hand I have come across many men and women who had indulged in excessive autoerotic and heterosexual practices and yet are potent even at a ripe old age...

"Masturbation itself is harmless, even if practiced to excess it does not produce insanity, or any nervous disorder or sexual weakness... *I have not come across a single case* (and I see many such cases in a year) *that can be directly attributed to masturbation."*

He further writes in answer to the question: how often do boys usually masturbate? "That varies, some a dozen times a month, and I have also known boys who have masturbated about a dozen times a day." Then again in answer to the question whether such constant loss of semen would not cause weakness in the body, he writes, . it does as little harm as, say, the loss of saliva.

Dr. Clifford Allen, M.D., M.R.C.P., D.P.M., author of several books writes in his book *Sexual Perversions and Abnormalities:* "There has been a great deal of misconception about masturbation in the past. It is worthwhile here examining the view that masturbation is harmful physically and psychically. Firstly from the physical point of view: The genitalia (Sex organs) consist of penis and testicles. These are activated by the nervous system. Does anyone of these organs become damaged by masturbation? The penis is piece of muscle. Now, we know that muscle, far from being injured by exercise, is improved. The penis is no exception, so that rather than injuring it, masturbation should make it stronger and more virile. Again, testicles are glands and the use does not injure a gland, except to make it hypertrophy (enlarged)... We can conclude with some reason that masturbation does not injure testicles. Does it injure the nervous system? This seems improbable since it is almost inexhaustible as a reflex center. Numerous physiologists have shown that it is impossible to exhaust a normal nerve fiber. It is impossible to damage the sexual organs by use...

"We might then ask the paradoxical question: 'Does masturbation have any useful functions?' One might produce a good case for the fact that it has a useful function. We know that misuse causes atrophy (degeneration). Every other muscle and gland in the body tends to atrophy if it is not used. Why should the genital organs from the exception? The truth is, however, that they are never allowed to atrophy. If the individual is deprived of normal sexual outlets, sexual urges arise which drive him to utilize his sexual organs in abnormal directions, the chief of which is masturbation. It may be that this is to preserve the integrity (health) of the sexual organs, until they can be used normally."

Dr. William S. Sadler, M.D., F.A.P.A., author of 3 books and having 50 years' experience, says in his book *practice of Psychiatry* "In almost 50 years of the practice of medicine I have yet to see a single real case where masturbation has been definitely responsible for ill health of any sort... Even yet the idea persists in the minds of a very considerable part of population that masturbation is in some way harmful to health. The time has come frankly to recognize that masturbation is not directly harmful to the physical health.. It in no way affects the health except through the worry over its supposed harmfulness or sinfulness... Masturbation, provided it is indulged without fear or moral regret, may, and often does, become a veritable health practice in that it directly relieves the physical sex tension."

Dr. Harold S. Diehl, M.A., M.D., D.Sc., Professor of Medicine, writes in his book *healthful Living:* "Masturbation is said to be an almost universal practice among healthy boys and common among girls... About 92 per cent of male college students admit masturbation, with the practice seemingly most common among healthy and robust athletes. In the more studious but physically less well-developed types it may occur frequently or only at rare intervals. Physically the habit, as ordinarily practiced, seems to be perfectly harmless... It is important that adolescent boys know that it is a harmless practice... it is always dangerous to warn boys against masturbation, even if the warning is a mild one, for they are apt to infer more than is said to them and to attribute to it all of their little failures and inadequacies until it becomes a really serious problem."

Dr. Hannah, M.D. and Dr. Abraham Stone, M.D., Write in their book *Marriage manual,* "Masturbation has been found to be fairly common sexual practice in nearly all human societies... There is certainly no evidence that it leads to physical injury or bodily harm... Any ill effects that may follow masturbation are due to the feelings of anxiety, guilt and self-condemnation, which it may bring about. Fear of consequences of masturbation is one of the most common sexual anxieties and constitutes an important sexual problem.

Dr. Havelock Ellis, the great sexologist and author of several books, writes in his book *Studies In the Psychology of Sex*: "At one time it (masturbation) was looked upon as a deadly sin leading to the most deadly consequences... A great deal of non-sense has been written about this subject. There are few healthy males who have not masturbated at one time or another. It was also said that the fluid which was lost during an emission came directly from the nervous systems, that the practice would cause diseases, such as tuberculosis, and would even lead to impotence. It is hardly necessary to point out that *there is no truth whatever in such assertions* (statements). One would think that it was scarcely worth mentioning these points now-a-days were it not for the fact that there still seem to be many people who believe them to be true." He means that now the harmlessness of masturbation is so clear that it may seem unnecessary to mention it, but he mentions it because so many people still believe that masturbation can cause harm. He further writes: "...it (masturbation) is also, in the absence of normal sexual relations, frequently not without good results. Masturbation is in the main, practiced for its sedative (soothing) effect on the nervous system..."

Dr. Norman Haire, the famous author and distinguished surgeon and doctor, writes in a note in the *Encyclopedia of Sexual Knowledge,* "Masturbation is a normal phenomenon which appears in a vast majority of children as well as in the young adults who are, for one reason or another, unable to obtain the normal satisfaction (by intercourse) of their sexual appetite, after they have become sexually mature. In adult life masturbation offers such poor satisfaction in comparison with normal sexual intercourse, that no normal healthy adult would practice it except when sexual intercourse is not available." He means that masturbation is normal and natural in those men who cannot have intercourse.

Dr. Marry Denham, author of several books on sex, writes in her book *Modern Views on Sex*: "Masturbation is almost universal in human race and not uncommon in animals. The modern view is to regard it as a normal manifestation. The older attitude of condemning masturbation as being an essentially harmful sexual perversion, an attitude that persists even today in certain types of moralists, has been productive of much harm. There is no justification for the statement that masturbation cause such serious physical weakness as may lead to nervous prostration, mental impairment and insanity... Where for various reasons marriage is delayed for many years after sexual maturity has been reached, masturbation in moderation means relief from disturbing sexual tension. It may be the only possible solution of the immediate sexual problem in certain circumstances."

Then she further writes on another page, "Probably the majority of adults who are leading celibate life resort to masturbation occasionally to relieve periodic sexual tension. A condition of celibacy (Brahmacharya) is unnatural for adults who are normally sexed."

Dr. Edwin W. Hirsch, M.D., sex specialist doctor and author of several books on sex, says in his book *Modern Sex Life*: "One of the biggest bugbears (Frightening things) which young men have to meet is the problem of masturbation. Most men at some time or another have indulged in self-gratification. Experienced physicians look upon the process of auto-erotism (masturbation) as a natural occurrence."

Dr. R.G. Gordon, M.D., D.Sc., F.R.C.S, author of several books, writes, "Masturbation must therefore be regarded as a way of satisfying the newly enforced impulse of sex, which is so insistent immediately after puberty. This practice in some form or at sometime is much more widespread than many people are willing to admit, and physically it cannot be said to do more harm than ordinary sexual intercourse."

Dr. W Stekel, M.D., author of the book *Impotence in the Male* in 2 volumes and over a dozen other similar big books, writes in this book: *"Masturbation is never the cause of impotence* (His italics). Unfortunately there are popular and pseudo-scientific books, which help to spread the false notion that masturbation causes impotence. I could mention hundreds of such misleading books. Practically every weak I see a victim of such literature on masturbation (*i.e.*, people who have come to believe themselves impotent by reading such misleading books.)...

"Whoever shows strong sexuality at an early age, in spite of masturbation and so-called sexual excesses, will preserve it to an advanced age." So many other similar extracts may be quoted from the books of this sexologist. He writes about himself.

"One of my comrades passed to me a book entitled *How to keep healthy*. The consequences of masturbation and of the loss of semen were described in it in a light that was more than terrifying. What horrible sufferings lay in store for the poor wretches who fell victim to this 'terrible crime.'? (Naturally I did not know at that time how common masturbation was among the young people.)

"The reading of this book caused me to pass through a serious mental crisis. Thanks to my robust constitution and my healthy mind that I was in the end none the worse for it.

"Nevertheless I repeat that the reading of that book had a most devastating effect on me. I was at that time passing through an important period of mental development. The verses I had written gave me the illusion of being a great poet. I loved nature and enjoyed looking at it. A sunrise would make me weep with emotion. But my health was, as I thought after reading that book, ruined forever, and this horrible idea upset me completely.

"Soon I experienced my first wet dreams and anxiety occasioned by this catastrophic' event with its loss of semen, haunted me irresistibly, and caused me to develop real hypochondria (a mental disorder by which a person wrongly believes that he is suffering from diseases, and worries for his health day and night).

"I rushed off to doctors to get myself examined. I read a number of books; but all that merely added to my anxiety, especially none of the practitioners I consulted seemed to understand me. The spectre of masturbation and its so-called after-effects hunted me up to consult the great scientific and medical authorities of the time. But they only treated me with probings and electricity, with water and with bromide..."

He then tells how he was relieved of his anxieties by consulting one of his professors who told him that masturbation had not harmed him in the least, and that one wet dream per week might be considered perfectly normal in youth.

Up to the 19th century in Europe also all people took a religious view of sex life according to which celibacy (Brahmacharya) is praised to the skies and sexual indulgence is regarded as bad and harmful; but in the 20th century with the advance of science when the scientific view of sex life was developed, it was realized that masturbation is natural in educated young men when they cannot have intercourse, and all medical and other scientific authorities (in Europe, America and India) are agreed on this fact. There are hundreds of scientific books on sex and health, and not a single one of them says that masturbation is harmful to the sex organs or general health. You can see such scientific books written by doctors in any good library. If you still go on believing and saying, "masturbation has ruined me," it would be very foolish of you. Some of the young men go on saying such foolish things, because worries and fears about masturbation continued for years have disturbed their minds seriously and made them rather insane or crazy in this matter. Try hard to remove such foolish beliefs and fears, which started in ignorance and became deep-rooted, strong and systematized as years went on, so that in course of time such beliefs and fears became a part of personality.

Self-healing Power of the Body. We may also consider the matter from the biological point of view. The bodies of all animals and men have a wonderful capacity of self-healing (of injuries), of endurance and recouping if weakened by starvation or disease, so why should the sex organs not heal themselves even if injured by masturbation? You see how our bodies repair even major injuries; limbs torn by tigers heal, and so also sword-cuts and bullet-wounds of battles. Medicines like penicillin which are applied to these wounds are only for killing the other living germs which enter the open wounds from the air, water and other things touching the wounds. It is these foreign invading germs that cause swelling and pus in the wounds (by eating the flesh) and thus prevent them from healing. Medicines only kill the germs they have no healing power as laymen believe. The healing is done by the body itself under the control and guidance of the brain. When tissues (flesh, bones etc.) are torn or broken without injuring the skin, which prevents the germs from entering the body, such internal injuries (as often caused by our falling from a tree etc.) are healed without any medicine. Thus when even bones are broken by a fall but the outer skin is unbroken and intact, the surgeons do nothing except putting the broken bone in the right straight position and fixing it there and giving complete rest (no medicines are applied). In a few days the broken bones become whole again by the body's self-healing power.

Then take the case of our body's recouping power in case of weakness by starving. If no food is given, your body can remain alive for about 2 months. For its working it would use the flesh from those muscles which are not so necessary, so that the body would remain almost a skeleton. The most essential organs (as brain, heart etc.) would be allowed to suffer last. And all this happens under the supervision of the brain, which is the most important organ of the body; other organs and systems of organs are in a way, merely tools of the brain, which it uses to keep itself alive and to reproduce other brains like itself. The brain uses the sexual system mainly for this purpose. Then when given food again after long starvation, the body builds itself again under the supervision of the brain and regains fully its normal weight, health and strength.

Then take recouping after a disease. Suppose a man suffers from a serious disease like typhoid fever, which is caused by some poisonous germs entering the body with food or water. The body would begin to fight with the invading germs so that every cell of it would take part in this struggle, which would go on constantly for over 3 weeks under high fever. During this emergency period there would be no sex desire or even hunger as, the brain does not want the body to spend its energy in sexual activities and in digesting food. The body (guided by lower brain) would use its own flesh (fat for its necessary working and fighting, so that by the end of the struggle it would be reduced to a skeleton.

Then after the germs are destroyed, the body takes rest, and then begins to build itself up again. It develops hunger again, which grows more and more as it gains strength to digest more and more food, and soon it begins to digest large amounts of food, as it never did normally. As the body regains its strength the sex desire also returns (after hunger and good digestion). Thus soon the extremely weakened body regains its normal weight, health and strength, then the increased hunger also returns to the normal. So such is the self-healing, recouping and self-regulating power of the body under the guidance of lower automatic centers of the brain.

Self-healing Power of the Sex Organs. In the sexual system also the body shows similar self-healing, recouping and self-regulating power. The woman's womb grows 200 times larger in advanced pregnancy (excluding the child and other contents). The vagina is badly torn in childbirth in many cases, yet it soon heals itself. In case of male organs also, when they are wounded or cut by accidents or in war time fighting, they heal similarly. In many cases of venereal diseases (gonorrhea, syphilis etc.) operations are performed on the penis and testicles and the diseased portions are cut off with a surgical knife. Again these wounds heal like other bodily wounds. Even the penis from which a good-sized portion is cut off from the top or the sides heals and has erection all right. Dr. Kenneth Walker, a great surgeon, sex specialist and author of the book *Sexual Disorders in the Male,* Writes in his book that it is surprising to see what remaining short and deformed penis is still capable of erection and intercourse after such mutilating operations or injuries due to war conditions or other such violent accidents.

Thus you see our body heals the bullet-wounds and swords-cuts and it also heals the injuries to the sex organs similarly. So, is it not foolish to believe that masturbation injures the sex organs so that the injury instead of being healed, grows more and more serious as time goes on and that gradually the man becomes impotent? It is all a childish belief caused by fear of impotence. In fact fear causes misbeliefs and guides their course, how misbeliefs arise out of the feeling of the feeling of fear as leaves arise out of branch. All your beliefs that masturbation had harmed you have arisen out of this fear, and this fear is usually aroused by the teaching of Brahmacharya in some form.

We may consider another biological principle. In higher animals and men (having good nervous systems) whenever the body is being injured or hurt by some activity, it feels pains and discomfort which is a warning of Nature that the man or animal stop activity. Even a sleeping animal would jump up and run away if you prick it with a small pin. Another natural sign of injury is continuous pain and swelling. No such thing happens in masturbation or intercourse. It is a certain proof that there is no injury. Only the foolish and ignorant people believe as if the penis is made of wax that it would be deformed or injured by such pleasant use as masturbation and intercourse.

Thus considered in any way, the belief that masturbation causes an injury, that the injury is permanent and ever increasing, is foolish, and this belief is caused by fear only, like the belief of ghosts. Only the utterly ignorant people have a fear and belief that as a result of masturbation a sort of ghost has entered their body and has started ruining it systematically.

Old School: From time immemorial masturbation has been considered as a very filthy habit and all sorts of ill effects have been attributed to it. The hard friction of hand makes the nerves of the glans very sensitive, and its hypersensitivity causes premature ejaculation so much so the boy gets discharged even after two or three strokes. If masturbation is practiced for more longer period the boy after marriage cannot make penetration and gets discharged outside the vaginal introitus. When the boy realizes the ill-effects of masturbation, he tries to stop this fility habit but as the whole system is hypersensitive he starts having very frequent night dreams. If it occur once or twice a month, they should be considered as mainly a phenomenon of male adolecence. But those boys who have masturbated excessively get wet dreams once or twice a week and sometime on alternate days. Some unfortunate victims get them daily. Excessive indulgence in masturbation next causes premature ejaculation. The boy discharges in four or five strokes, afterwards impotence ushers in. The boy gets very weak erections or they fail to develop. At this stage the boy is completely a sexual wreck and impotent.

Excessive masturbation: Some people say that ordinarily masturbation may be harmless, but if practised excessively, only then it may cause harm. Of course this view is correct and true. As we all know the saying "Excess of everything is bad" This saying aptly applicable over masturbation also. We can understand simply by taking an example. Excessive eating leads to indigestion resulting in loss of appetite, gas formation, acidity or loose motions. Similarly excessive masterbaution may cause damage to nerve endings of the glans penis making them hypersensitive so that impulses from glans are carried to the brain in very rapid succession and the point of ejaculation is reached at very rapid pace and the semen is discharged very quickly. Therefore the first wrong caused by excessive masturbation is "Premature ejaculation".

Secondly by indulging excessively in the self-erotic process the various centers and the organs related with sexual activity get exhausted and their normal functioning such as erection is affected and the victim faces loss of libido or loss of erection.

Thus the very thing done in moderation causes no harm (What the Kinsey & others meant) proves disastrous and brings in it's wake catastrophe such as Quick emissions, complete or partial loss of erection and of course with little desire for sexual activity, if indulged in excessively.

Therefore young boys are advised not to be misguided by the advice of Kinsey and others and should not indulge in masturbation excessively. Kinsey and others are correct but it should be remembered they never meant excessive indulgence. It is certain, if masturbation would be indulged in excessively it may jeopardize the future sex life of the youth or the adolescent beyond recovery.

Author's view: In my opinion the middle course is best. First of all one should avoid masturbation altogether because masturbation is habit forming process and one is liable to go for it in excess. As the alcohol, opium and other narcotic drugs are habit forming so is masturbation. Therefore I would like to advise younger generation to avoid it altogether so that it does not become one's part of life. Secondly if it has been practiced in the past, one should not feel guiltily about it because masturbation done sparingly leaves no scar and cause no harm. Only guilt feeling or repentance would affect the victim emotionally.

I am sure, the readers would take the findings of Kinsey and others in right perspective and never indulge in masturbation excessively. I advise to avoid it all together and as you know when one is addicted to anything may be–it is alcohol or opium–one is bound to go in for excesses.

The last warning. Young boys! If you are indulging in masturbation excessively you are certainly jeopardizing your future. Therefore stop it completely and perhaps this is the right time. If you feel some sort of weakness or debility certainly take advice of a sex specialist and go for treatment as directed by him.

Chapter-4

The Clitoris – Woman's Mysterious Sex Organ

The GERMANS call it "the tickler".

The English call it "the man in the boat".

The Arabs and Africans often amputate it.

A good many do not even know that it exists.

I refer to the clitoris, the female sex organ that is so little known to the average man that it is a source of complete mystery. And that is greatly to be regretted, because it is difficult and sometimes almost impossible to give a woman sexual satisfaction without understanding the role that the clitoris plays.

The clitoris has almost always been misunderstood – so much, so that even its scientific name is an inaccurate one, if the philologists are correct. It is derived from a Greek work, *kleitoris*, which is simply the Greek name of the organ in question. But *kleitoris*, in turn, is thought to derive from the Greek word *kleiein*, which means, "to shut"– as though the clitoris could possibly shut or bar the entrance to the vagina, an anatomic improbability.

What is the clitoris, and why is it so important in the sexual relation?

The clitoris is the female equivalent of the penis, anatomically speaking. It is a miniature penis in many respects, having a shaft; a glans; or head; a prepuce, or foreskin; and the ability to become erect during sexual excitement.

The clitoris is small – about the size of a small pea, usually. But its size can vary greatly from woman to woman. The gynecologist R.L. Dickinson examined 100 women, measuring their clitorises, and found that in 5 percent the organ was two–sixteenth of an inch in height, in 75 percent it was between two–sixteenth and one–fourth of an inch, in 20 percent it was from five–sixteenth to one–half an inch. As we will see in a moment, there are cases on record in which the clitoris is much larger even than that.

It is an organ richly supplied with nerves that has an elaborate network of tiny blood vessels. When stimulated by contact or by general sexual arousal, these blood vessels begin to fill, the clitoris swell. When erect, it can be as much as twice the size of its normal state. Also, during an erection of the clitoris, the foreskin draws back, exposing the highly sensitive glans, so that even more vivid stimulation becomes possible.

The clitoris is located within the vulva, or external female genitals. The most conspicuous features of the vulva are the *labia majora,* or outer lips. Within these are the *labia minora,* or inner lips, which are usually not visible except when the outer lips are parted. Hidden within these inner lips is the entrance to the vagina. Just above the vaginal opening is the meatus; or external opening of the urinary tract. The clitoris is located above the meatus and within the inner lips.

The placement of the clitoris is vital to a women's sexual happiness. For the clitoris is probably the chief center of sexual excitement. It is much more richly endowed with nerves than the vagina, for instance. The thrusts of the penis into the vagina conveys relatively little stimulation to a woman, compared with the excitement that is produced when the penis rubs against the clitoris on each of its strokes.

But if the clitoris is situated too high within the lips, the penis will not normally come in contact with it at all.

Usually, the clitoris is an inch and a half or less above the meatus, M.M. Bolles and C. Landis, in their 1942 study, measured the clitoris–meatus distance in several hundred women and concluded that when the clitoris was more than an inch and a half above the meatus, sexual pleasure was difficult for a woman to obtain.

There are two ways for the clitoris to be stimulated during intercourse – by contact with the upper surface of the penis as it rhythmically penetrates the vagina, and by the pressure of the pubic area of the male against the organ. But in many instances the clitoris is so placed that the even this pressure is not felt.

Since the clitoris is obviously so important in the female sexual response, how is it that many men have no knowledge of it all? They wouldn't attempt to drive a car without knowing where the accelator is. How can they go to bed with a woman without being aware of the "master organ" of female sensuality?

Sheer ignorance is part of the answer. No one has told them that the clitoris is there, and they don't have enough curiosity to find out.

Prudishness is another part of the explanation: Male prudishness keeps many men from *looking* at the female genital region. As one man, a clerk with little education, expressed it, "It's ugly, I don't like to look at it. I just like to get inside it". Female prudishness figures into the problem also, since many women who are very well aware of the existence and importance of the clitoris are too shy to call it to their husbands' attention.

Finally, the clitoris is extremely small. As we have seen, in some women it is less than one-eighth of an inch in length. Extremely fleshy women may be so plump that the clitoris can't be seen within the inner lips. In few women, the clitoris is "hooded" by a flap of skin, which not only hides it from sight but also effectively shields it from any sort of pleasurable stimulation. Such women are usually frigid, though the "hood" of the clitoris can be removed in a simple surgical operation once the existence of the condition is discovered.

However, the clitoris is not always so tiny that it is difficult to see. The annals of medical history bulge with strange cases of enlarged clitoris, in which the organ often takes on the appearance of a true penis. Many of them so-called hermaphrodites–double-sexed individuals who seem to have female breasts but male sex organs – are actually women with greatly enlarged clitorises.

In the classic nineteenth-century volume *Anomalies and Curiosities of Medicine,* by Drs. George M. Gould and Walter M. Pyle, we are given some of the famous cases of this sort recorded in the past.

> *Otto at Breslau in 1824 reports seeing a negress with a clitoris 4½ inches long and 1½ inches in the transverse diameter; it projected from the vulva and when supine formed a complete covering for a vaginal orifice. (In such freak cases the original Greek meaning of the word does have some justification).*
>
> *The clitoris may at times become so large so to prevent coitus.*
>
> *Columbus cites an example of a clitoris as long as a little finger; Hailer mentions one which measured seven inches, and there is a record of an enlarged clitoris which resembled the neck of a goose and which was 12 inches long.*

The enlarged clitoris appears to be a racial trait among the peoples of North Africa. However, this does not mean that the women of Egypt or Morocco or Tunisia have been abnormally sensitive to sexual stimulation– because in various African countries there has long been practiced the cruel and barbaric custom of *clitoridectomy,* aptly called "The sexual crippling of women".

Clitoridectomy is the amputation of the clitoris. In some tribes it is performed at the age of puberty. Since it removes the center of sensual nervous stimulation in a woman, it effectively destroys much of her ability to receive pleasure in the act of love.

In certain areas, circumcision of the clitoris is performed instead of clitoridectomy. This is a painful and terrifying experience, performed without anesthetics and with crude knives, but it is not quite so cruel as the complete removal of the organ.

In their study of Afro–Asian sexuality, *The Cradle of Erotica,* Allen Edwardes and R.E.L. Masters provide this grim description of clitoridectomy in the Arab lands.

> *For clitoridectomy, the little child is seated with her thighs held wide apart by the surgeon's assistant. Then the surgeon, generally a skillful if formally uneducated woman, seizes hold of the protruding clitoris with her thumb and forefinger and pinches or pulls it until it stiffens;*

> *stiffens; whereupon she slices it off with a single stroke of the razor. If the clitoris is concealed within the labial folds, the surgeon will make a shallow incision or cut away the prepuce to expose the glans.*

When the clitoris is merely circumcised, baring the glans, sexual sensitivity is actually increased. But more often the operation is a clitoridectomy – reducing the woman to the state of a sexual cripple. The theory is that by removing the clitoris, the vagina will become more sensitive to stimulation. This is perhaps true in some cases. In many, surgical frigidity is the chief result.

Even so, the custom is ingrained, and the women do not seem to object to it. To call a girl of the Sudan "Un–circumcised" is like calling her a slut – a high insult. In ancient Egypt, a woman who had not been circumcised did not have full legal rights and could not own property, for example.

Ask any ten men at random to identify the clitoris, and it is quite likely that seven of them will not know what you are talking about. If you choose your ten men from the lower educational levels of society, you are quite likely to get a ten–out–of–ten "don't know" response. Even if you simply ask men to describe the external appearance of the female genitals, you will find most if not all of them failing to mention the clitoris.

If they know it is there at all, they generally don't realize how important it is to the sexual stimulation of the female. They regard the vagina, not the clitoris, as the center of physical excitement for a woman.

Even the authorities are in some disagreement about the relative importance of the clitoris and the vagina in sexual intercourse. Sigmudn Freud believed that the clitoris was important only in childhood and that as a woman matured she transferred the center of her receptivity from the clitoris to the vagina, except in cases of neurosis. Freud wrote in *A General Introduction of Psychoanalysis.*

> *The clitoris in the girl, moreover, is in every way equivalent to the penis. It is a region of especial excitability in which autoerotic satisfaction (masterbation) is achieved. In the transition to womanhood very much depends on the early and complete relegation of this*

> *sensitivity from the clitoris over to the vaginal orifice. In those women who are sexually anesthetic, as it is called (frigid, that is), the clitoris has stubbornly retained this sensitivity.*

Freud's theory about the clitoris is still held by some of his most orthodox supporters. Most competent sexologists today, however, believe that it is quite normal for the clitoris to remain the center of sexual excitation for a woman and doubt that the vagina is really as sensitive.

The clitoris, then, is of prime importance in the sexual life of women. Any man who considers himself a sophisticated lover must develop knowledge of the clitoris's role and a mastery of the arts of stimulating it in foreplay. For there must be a good deal of attention paid to the clitoris before penetration takes place. In nearly all women except the most passionate, full culmination is impossible without prolonged precoital caresses of the clitoris.

The story is told of the one-time Empress of Austria who was bothered by frigidity. The royal physician examined Her Majesty, heard her complaints of sterility and sexual dissatisfaction, and delivered a famous opinion that deserves to be engraved on the wall of every bedroom in the country.

"I am of the opinion," he declared, "that the sexual organs of Your Most Sacred Majesty should be titillated for some considerable time before coitus".

This titillation, of course, should be carried out by the husband with the same delicacy and care that is necessary in any other phase of the act. It should be done infinitely lightly, since this organ is incredibly sensitive. With a light touch of the fingertip, the lover strokes and caresses the tiny organ, which will swell and throb with excitement. The foreskin will pull back, exposing the highly sensitive glans, or head of the clitoris, and this should be touched even more delicately. Soft words of love, and the stroking or kissing on the breasts and nipples, will add to the voluptuousness of the sensations for the woman, bringing her closer and closer to that moment of receptivity when the penis can be plunged into the warm, moist depths of the vagina.

Thus the clitoris becomes the center of attention as the foreplay reaches its climax. Despite this, a vast number of husbands pay no attention to it and concentrate simply on entering the vagina – in complete ignorance of the true mechanism of female sensuality.

There are some women, however, who are exceptions to the general rule. They do not like direct stimulation applied to the clitoris. There are several possible reasons for this attitude.

A small minority of women have ultrasensitive clitorises. They cannot bear to have them touched. In such cases, this element of foreplay must be omitted, and it may even be necessary to avoid those positions of intercourse, which apply too much pressure to the clitoris. Women of this sort are generally frigid, though sometimes their vaginas are also abnormally sensitive and they can be brought to climax through vaginal stimulation without any contact with the clitoris whatever.

There is also a neurotic fear of having the clitoris touched, usually stemming from the fact that the woman is habitually given to masturbation. Contrary to popular male belief, most women do not masturbate by inserting objects such as candles into their vaginas. Rather, they stimulate their clitorises with their fingers until they reach orgasm.

If a woman is a regular clitoridal masturbator and has serious guilt feelings about this practice, she may object when her husband attempts to manipulate her clitoris. It will seem too clear a reminder of her own secret practice. Her feelings of guilt will not allow her to accept a caress that she has come to regard as "shameful".

However, in most instances women welcome stimulation of the clitoris – provided it is applied with a light touch. It is an invaluable form of foreplay. It may also be used in what can called "afterplay" to complete a sex act that might otherwise end unsatisfactorily for the woman.

For example, even the most virile of men occasionally suffers the embarrassment of a premature ejaculation. He reaches his orgasm too soon with his wife still one to five minutes away from her fulfillment. Very often, the penis will go limp soon after the male orgasm. It thus becomes impossible to continue intercourse. The considerate and skilled husband, however, will use clitoridal afterplay. By stroking his wife's clitoris, he will bring her on to her orgasm. The alternative is to leave her dissatisfied and tense – as many prematurely ejaculating husbands are content to do.

Thus in short, clitoris is the key to sexual success. There is no excuse for ignorance of this vital organ.

Chapter-5

The G-Spot

Three times in this century, great pioneers in the field of human sexuality have shocked, informed, and transformed our world. The people responsible for these seismic changes are Sigmund Freud, Alfred Kinsey and his co-workers, and the team of Masters and Johnson. They influenced us in far more significant ways than many of us may realize. Their works has significantly shaped our attitudes, influenced our behaviour, and changed our lives in many ways; however, their findings and their theoretical conclusions contradict each other, which leaves us in a very real dilemma. **Freud** told us that the mature woman is vaginally responsive and should give up her childish interest in her clitoris. **Kinsey** and co-workers, and more recently **Masters and Johnson**, assured us that orgasm in all women involves the clitoris and that it is the main focus of female erotic arousal.

Freud was born in what is now Czechoslovakia, in 1856, just sixteen years after Queen Victoria married her beloved Albert. Freud's family moved to Vienna when he was four years old and his entire education took place in that great cultural center. In order to support his wife and children he gave us a career in laboratory research and became a neurologist in private practice. He saw the clitoris as a protruding 'masculine' organ, a vestigial, inferior penis. Being more accessible than the vagina, it is naturally discovered first by little girls in their play and self-exploration, Freud theorized that as a girl matures and becomes a woman, she must give up her childish interest in her clitoris and 'transfer' the focus of her pleasurable feelings to her vagina. (The vagina is a receptive organ and women are supposed to be receptive). This came to be known as the **clitoral-vaginal transfer theory.** Many of Freud's theories are accepted today as valid. In fact, he is regarded as one of the creative giants of all time, with good reason. But the fact is that Freud, in spite of his great contributions, made some significant errors.

It was not until the 1950s, when biologist Alfred Kinsey, Ph. D., began to study the sexual habits of men and women. One result of Kinsey's work was Freud's clitoral - vaginal transfer theory began to be officially challenged. There were, of course, millions of women all along who had experienced clitoral pleasure, but they hadn't said much about it publicly. He had collected more than 7,000 of the approximately 17,000 case histories that were completed at the time of his death. We learned a lot about human sexual behaviour from those interviews, which were far more comprehensive that any previously undertaken. In a lecture at the New York Academy of Medicine in 1955, shortly before Kinsey's death, a packed house filled with prestigious members of the medical profession heard Kinsey talk about the wide variety of male and female sexual behaviour. But as time went by it was generally accepted that, his data were the most reliable in existence. Like Freud, and all other great pioneers, Kinsey made some errors. In a special research project initiated by the Kinsey Institute an attempt was made to find out which areas of a woman's genitals are most sensitive to sexual stimulation. Three male and two female gynaecologists tested more than 800 women by touching sixteen points, including the clitoris labia (major and minor), vaginal lining, and cervix. Unfortunately, sensitive areas of the vagina, we now know, respond to deep pressure but not soft touch, and so the Kinsey researchers concluded, erroneously, that the clitoris is sensitive and the vagina is not.

Encouraged by the scientific progress made through Kinsey's pioneering work, Masters and Johnson took the final courageous step and decided to observe sex firsthand in the laboratory and then report their findings. All female orgasm, according to them, involves the clitoris and is physiologically indistinguishable. At the opposite end of the spectrum, Masters and Johnson's findings released a flood of literature extolling the virtues of the clitoris. Masters and Johnson's notion, however, that all orgasms involve the clitoris was not confirmed by the subjective experience of most of the respondents.

Three years later, in 1980, at the national meeting of the Society for the Scientific Study of Sex (SSSS), **John Perry** and **Beverly Whipple** opened new vistas and told the conference that:

- There is a spot inside the vagina that is extremely sensitive to deep pressure. It lies in the anterior wall of the vagina about two inches from the entrance. They named this area the Grafenberg spot, after Dr. Ernst Grafenberg, the first modern physician to describe it.
- The spot has been found in every woman they had examined.
- When properly stimulated, the Grafenberg spot swells and leads to orgasm in many women.
- At the moment of orgasm, many women ejaculate a liquid through the urethra that is chemically similar to male ejaculate but contains no sperm.
- As a result of stimulation of the G-spot, women often have a series of orgasms.
- For many women it is difficult to properly stimulate the G-spot in the missionary position. Other positions work better.
- Using a diaphragm for birth control interferes with stimulation of the G-spot in some women.
- Because they believe they are urinating, many women are embarrassed about ejaculating. Thinking the same thing, their partners often belittle them, which is one reason many women have learned to suppress orgasm.
- The strength of a woman's pubococcygeus muscle is directly related to her ability to reach orgasm through intercourse.
- Women can learn to strengthen their pubococcygeus muscles or to relax them if they are too tense.
- If men increase the strength of their pubococcygeus muscles, they too can learn to become multiply orgasmic and separate orgasm from ejaculation.
- There are several types of orgasm in women and men. In women there is a vulval orgasm, triggered by the clitoris a

uterine orgasm, triggered by intercourse, and a combination of the two. In men there is an orgasm triggered by the penis and one by the prostate.

Although this was not the first time that Perry and Whipple had presented their data, it was a historic moment in the field of sex research. After some time Dr. Martin Weisberg, M.D., a gynecologist at Thomas Jefferson University Hospital in Philadelphia accepted Perry and Whipple's above theory (who was reluctant before) and agreed that *The Vulva and vagina were normal with no abnormal masses or spots. The urethra was normal. Everything was normal. She then had her partner stimulate her by inserting two fingers into the vagina and stroking along the urethra lengthwise. To our amazement, the area began to swell. It eventually became a firm one by two cm oval area distinctly different from the rest of the vagina. And seconds later several cc's of milky fluid shot out of the urethra. The material was clearly not urine. In fact, if the chemical analysis described in the paper is correct, its composition was closest of prostatic fluid. A few patients of mine told me that they ejaculate. Some about erotic area around urethra known. And everyone who went home to experiment found the* ***Grafenberg spot.*** *In the end he added that in his opinion Grafenberg spot and female ejaculation exist.*

People at the SSSS meeting seemed very excited about Perry and Whipple's report. Especially about the Grafenberg spot and different type of female orgasm. These four discoveries, Grafenberg spot, female ejaculation, the importance of pelvic muscle and the continuum of orgasmic response, unify the findings of the Freudians and other sex researchers into an understandable and consistent whole. We now have a new synthesis that validates the experience of both vaginal and clitoral orgasm. **In short Grafenberg spot is a** *magic spot* **and tops the erotic zones of females.**

Where exactly is the G-spot located? The Grafenberg spot lies directly behind the pubic bone within the front wall of the vagina. It is usually located about halfway between the back of the pubic bone and the front of the cervix, along the course of the urethra (the tube through which female urinate) and near the neck of the bladder, where it connects with the urethra. The size and exact location vary. (Imagine a small clock inside the vagina with 12 O'clock pointing towards the navel. The majority of women will find the G-spot located in the area between 11 and 10 O'clock). Unlike the clitoris, which profrudes from the surrounding tissue, it lies deep within the vaginal wall, and a firm pressure is often needed to contact the G-spot in its unstimulated state.

We first read about the existence of this sensitive area in the anterior wall of the vagina from an article written by Graffeberg in 1950, in which he said:

.... an erotic zone could always be demonstrated on the anterior wall of the vagina along the course of the urethra .... (which) seems to be surrounded by erectile tissue like the Corpora Cavernosa (of the penis).... In the course of sexual stimulation, the female urethra begins to enlarge and can be easily felt. It swells out greatly at the end of the orgasm. The most stimulating part is located at the posterior urethra, where it arises from the neck of the bladder.

Grafenberg did not dispute Kinsey's findings about the clitoris, but he did insist that the vagina was also important. Because of his clear descriptions of the relationship of a sensitive area in the vagina to sexual pleasure, Perry and Whipple named this area - the *Grafenberg spot*.

Chapter-6

Drugs and Their Negative Sexual Effects

A very little section of people know that a wide range of drugs affect sexual functioning. It is possible that any drug you are taking for the treatment of hypertension (High Blood Pressure), heart disease, anxiety or stress, depression, psychiatric illness, sleeplessness, convulsions, gastrointestinal disorders, or arthritis may affect your sexual functioning. Some times it can take several years before a medication causes sexual side effects. Therefore if you develop a sexual dysfunction while being treated with a medication, go to your physician and tell him or her about symptoms. Together your work to discover whether it is the medication, some aspect of your illness, or something else in your life that is causing the dysfunction. Once the cause is identified, help is available to resolve the sexual difficulty.

Common sense would suggest that a physician would tell patient in advance about potential sex-related side effects, but often they don't. Some physicians do not because they believe that it will lead to anxiety about sexual functioning, which itself can result in dysfunction. However, a patient who does not know in advance about the possibility of such side effects may assume that any sexual problem is an inevitable sign of aging or an unavoidable consequence of the disease. As result the patient doesn't seek a solution.

If you suspect that a medication has affected your sex life, talk to your physician. Ask if you can try a different dosage or another drug. No one should be embarrassed to mention sexual difficulties to a doctor or to ask to solution. If your physician seems unwilling to help you, find one who will.

Unfortunately, solving problems with the sexual side effects of drugs is a trial-and-error process. One difficulty is the same medication can affect individuals differently. Therefore, finding out whether a problem is due to a medication or some other physical or psychological factor is difficult and requires cooperation and patience on the part of both physician and patient. Once you a found a physician who is willing to work with you, stick with him or her until the problem has been solved regardless of how long it takes. *But do not experiment on your own; reducing or stopping medication can jeopardize your health.* Even if sexual problems appear and if takes sometime to diagnose and resolve them, do not assume your sex life is over. While you are working on finding a solution, there are sexual activities, which can provide satisfaction. For example, if a man does not have erections, often he can still have pleasurable ejaculation and orgasm. There are many sexual activities that can provide satisfying orgasms for both partners. Above all, continue to exchange affection with your partner.

The generic drugs listed below are capable of affecting some aspects of sexuality. Your physician or pharmacist will be able to tell you the brand names under which these drugs are marketed if you do not know them. As would be expected, the principal therapeutic effect of all of them is on the nervous or circulatory systems. As with any drug effect, the nature and degree of altered sexual function will vary greatly from one individual to another. While such effects may occur at any age, they are usually more frequent and more troublesome after the age of fifty. If you suspect the possibility of such a drug response, consult your physician regarding the advisability of modifying your treatment program.

Drug name or family	***Possible effects***
Alcohol	Reduced potency in men, delayed orgasm in Women.
Amphetamine	Reduced libido and potency.
Bethanidine	Impaired ejaculation.
Clonidine	Reduced libido.
Debrisoquine	Reduced potency, impaired ejaculation.
Dextroamphetamine	Reduced libido and potency, impaired ejaculation.
Diazepam	Reduced desire, ejaculation problems and impaired orgasm.

Disulfiram	Reduced potency.
Guanethidine	Reduced potency, impaired ejaculation.
Haloperidol	Reduced potency.
Levodopa	Increased libido (in some men and women)
Lithium	Reduced potency.
Methyldopa	Reduced libido and potency.
Oral contraceptives	Reduced libido (in some women)
Phenothiazines	Reduced libido and potency, impaired ejaculation (occasionally)
Phenoxybenzamine	Impaired ejaculation.
Primidone	Reduced libido and potency.
Reserpine	Reduced libido and potency.
Sedative and sleep-inducing drugs (Hypnotics) when used on a regular Basis.	Reduced libido and potency.
Thiazide diuretics	Reduced libido (occasionally in some men).
Tranquilizers (mild)	Reduced libido and potency.
Tricyclic antidepressants	Reduced libido and potency.

The short list provided above represents only a few medications that may have an effect on your sexual functioning. Just because the name of your drug is not listed here dose not mean that it is not capable of producing negative sexual side-effects. Consult your doctor, if your particular drug has any adverse effect on sexuality.

When in doubt and you suspect your drug is effecting you adversely speak directly to your physician about adjusting dosage or changing to a different drug. If your physician is not helpful, consult some 'sexologist' who may be better informed and capable of solving your problem.

Chapter-7

Circumcision

Circumcision is the oldest as well as the most widely practiced surgical operation, and it is the only one that bears a mystical or religious significance. The operation consists in the removal of the foreskin—a double layer of skin and mucous membrane, which covers the glans penis more or less completely. In every male animal throughout Nature, the glans is thus covered, undoubtedly as a protective measure in Nature's economy.

Yet, since prehistoric times, circumcision has been practiced as a ritual by peoples unrelated and widely scattered over the face of the globe. Where the practice originated and why is still clouded in mystery. We know that the Egyptians practiced it at least 17 centuries B.C., and the Arabs at least 4 centuries B.C., while the Jews have practiced circumcision as a symbol of the Biblical covenant between God and Abraham for nearly 4000 years. Cortez found it practiced in Mexico and the practice was common among the Aztecs, the Mayas, some of the American Indian tribes, the aborigines of Australia and in South America along the Orinoco.

To-day circumcision is practiced ritually not only by the Jews and Mohammedans, but in many parts of the world; and it is a curious fact that certain primitive tribes which practice circumcision live alongside other tribes which do not adhere to this ritual. In Madagascar and other places, the boy's godfather eats the foreskin dipped in egg-yolk.

It is interesting to note that a similar operation, removing the foreskin, which covers the clitoris in the female, is also very widely practiced in Arabia, Egypt and other parts of Asia and Africa. In females the foreskin, which covers the clitoris, is removed. Some still believe that female circumcision has its own advantage and prevents them in indulging masturbation due to retained smegma or adherent prepuce.

As regards male circumcision, it must be obvious that this practice, which has such an ancient history and almost universal distribution and has survived these thousands of years with increasing popularity, must have something more than a merely ritualistic or racial basis to account for its survival and popularity in civilized life. This can be readily explained by considering the subject from a medical and hygienic standpoint. Circumcision has its ardent advocates as a hygienic measure but it also has strong opponents among medical men. Let us first consider the reasons given by those who oppose routine circumcision:

1, That Nature has endowed all male animals with a foreskin as a protective covering for the sensitive glans, and it is therefore a contravention of Nature to remove this protective covering; 2, That circumcision is a relic of barbarism, and as such should not be practiced by civilized peoples; 3, That removal of the foreskin deadens the nervous sensitiveness of the glans in the act of coitus, and thus diminishes sexual pleasure and predisposes to eventual impotence: 4, That the hygienic benefits ascribed to circumcision can be attained equally as well by various palliative measure, such as stretching, passing a probe around the preputial cavity, and a high degree of cleanliness.

These objections to circumcision are readily answered by its proponents as follows: 1, It is true that the foreskin offers protection to the sensitive glans in lower animals and undoubtedly served the same function for primitive man; but now that men wear clothes and do not live in jungles, the foreskin is entirely unnecessary as a protective organ; 2, while we are not concerned with the barbarous origin of circumcision, we are concerned with the fact that it offers many hygienic and prophylactic benefits of which we, as civilized men, should take advantage; 3, the charge that circumcision diminishes sexual sensitiveness and induces impotence is completely negative by the fact that the races and peoples who have practiced years are concededly among the most prolific and sexually virile peoples in the world and their sexual potency has never been questioned; 4, stretching the foreskin and passing the probe within its cavity may afford momentary relief in some cases with adhesions, but these measures never have been shown to be of permanent value; and lastly, the smegma and other accumulations within the preputial cavity absolutely preclude the possibility of a degree of genital cleanliness even comparable with that attained as the result of circumcision.

Having disposed of the objections to circumcision let us considers the definite advantages, which this operation performed in infancy offers. The writer, for many years, has advocated infantile circumcision purely as a hygienic measure. His reasons have been given in detail in previous publications to which the reader is referred. Briefly stated, these reasons are as follows:

1. In the circumcised there is no secretion of smegma and no accumulation of urine and other secretions, with the resultant absence of the odor, which so often clings to the uncircumcised, even to those who are familiar with soap and water. A certain degree of banalities is practically always present in the uncircumcised and no amount of washing and cleansing seems to be able to eradicate the secretions of the foreskin and their penetrating odor.

2. Phimosis and paraphimosis cannot occur in the circumcised. That is obvious. Consequently the pathologic conditions which follow in the wake of phimosis and paraphimosis cannot and do not occur in the circumcised. It may be mentioned as an interesting historical fact that the phimosis of Louis XVI, of France, and his consequent impotence which was finally relieved, seven years after his marriage, by circumcision, are held to be largely responsible for the excesses of his spouse Marie Antoinette, which undoubtedly helped to bring about the Revolution and the execution of the King and Queen.

3. Circumcision protects against syphilis and chancroid. The reasons are obvious. The foreskin is the favorite site for about 75 per cent of primary chancres and even a greater proportion of chancroids. Leading American authorities are practically unanimous in the opinion that syphilis and chancroid are much more common in the uncircumcised. It is obvious that it must be so because of the greater liability of infection in the unclean and constantly irritated tissues in the uncircumcised.

4. Circumcision is a 100 per cent prophylactic against cancer. Limitations of space forbid more than a brief statement of the

facts. It may be accepted as proven beyond the shadow of doubt that penis cancer has never been reported in a man circumcised in infancy, whereas this form of cancer constitutes from 2 to 3 per cent of all cancer in men.

It has been stated that the freedom from cancer among the Jews is racial in character. There can be no doubt that the recognized immunity of Jews against penis cancer is due entirely to the absence of the foreskin from the very earliest days of life. In other words, where there is no foreskin there will be no cancer.

5. Circumcision is a prophylactic against masturbation, convulsions in infants, and other reflex irritative phenomena. The literature abounds with evidence to corroborate this statement. The reader is referred to the writings of Gowers, Baker, Lydston, Moll and Block for details.

6. Circumcision is a prophylactic against local complications in venereal disease. Balanitis, with extensive ulceration and necrosis of the glans and foreskin may supervene in the presence of a long and tight foreskin. Suppurating adenitis (bubo) is far more common in chancroid and gonorrhea when a foreskin is present to dam the natural drainage of the pathologic secretions. The dorsal incision, so often necessary to liberate the accumulated debris and expose the original lesion to view, is but a poor substitute for circumcision.

7. In some cases of premature ejaculation circumcision has been considered of value in prolonging coitus since the uncovered glans may be somewhat less sensitive. Thus circumcision decreases the sensitivity of the glans and man is able to prolong the coitus for a longer time.

In conclusion, it must stated that circumcision is a most valuable hygienic measure and a great aid to personal cleanliness and prophylactic against many sexually transmitted diseases and helps to some degree in overcoming the distressing complaint called premature ejaculation.

Chapter-8

Sexually Transmitted Diseases (STDs)

There is no single disease called VD (Venereal Disease). In the past this phrase was a blanket classification that included all sexually transmitted diseases (STDs). Now more than 50 diseases are called STDs and each has its own different infectious organism, symptoms, tests, and treatment. These diseases can be uncomfortable or even painful, terribly inconvenient, embarrassing, and anxiety-producing. Some kill. They can be passed on to those we care most about—our wives, husbands, and lovers by having sex and to our offspring before they are born. Infection with the AIDS virus (Human Immunodeficiency Virus—HIV) leads to devastating illness and death in a large percentage of those infected. Human *papillomavirus* (HPV), which causes genital warts, appears to provide the first step in the development of genital cancers. Syphilis (now a curable disease if diagnosed and treated in its early stages) can lead after many years to paralysis, severe mental illness, and ultimately death if untreated.

Other STDs either never disappear or *leave damage* that is difficult or impossible to erase. Although not the scourge it was first thought to be, once the herpes virus enters the body it remains for the rest of a person's life and causes painful sores that can appear over and over again for many years. If not treated early enough, other STD organisms (like chlamydia and gonorrhea), often lead to Scarring of the reproductive tract. This can result in infertility and the risk of pregnancy in the Fallopian tubes (ectopic pregnancy), which results in internal bleeding sometimes death. Finally, many STDs can be transmitted from the mother to the fetus during pregnancy or delivery, often resulting in much more devastating and life-threatening illness in newborns than in adults.

I hope it is abundantly clear that any symptoms of genital infection must be immediately diagnosed and treated to protect both the infected individuals and their sexual partners. One of the problems in diagnosing STDs is that many different organism cause nearly identical symptoms.

Some Important Facts About STDs

· A large number of individuals who are infected with STDs experience *no* symptoms (this is called being asymptomatic). This is especially true for women who develop PID (Pelvic Inflammatory Disease), which can result in infertility without symptoms.

· Even if no symptoms are present, sexually active men and women should be tested for possible infection with the common (often asymptomatic) STDs during annual medical examinations. This is especially important for those individuals who are not in mutual sexually exclusive relationships and those who have changed partners since their last doctor's appointment.

· With respect to a number of STDs, women are at higher risk of becoming infected from *one* act of intercourse than are men.

· In general, women are more likely to be "receivers" and men are more likely to be "infectors." That is, women are more likely to catch STDs from men than men are from women.

· Douching to prevent STD infection is not effective and may increase the risk that a genital infection moves into the reproductive organs (PID) and leads to infertility.

· All STDs are treatable and most are curable *if* they are diagnosed and treated early.

· Women should *not* douche before any pelvic examination as this can hide symptoms and alter test results, making diagnosis of STDs difficult or impossible.

· When an STD is diagnosed, sexual partners should always be treated at the same time to avoid the ping-pong effect (passing the infection back and forth between partners).

Things One Can Do To Lower One's Risks

"Safer sex" guidelines were developed in response to the AIDS epidemic. However, these guidelines for protecting oneself from the AIDS virus (HIV) are just as effective at protecting you from other STD organisms. The reason these are called "safer" rather than "safe" is because they are not 100 percent guaranteed, but they clearly do reduce your risks *if* used properly and every time.

"Safer Sex" Guidelines

1. **Delay sexual intercourse as long as possible.** Abstinence is the only completely safe behaviour.

2. **Restrict the number of sexual partners you have.** The fewer sexual partners you have in your lifetime, the smaller your chance of being exposed to an STD.

3. **You are at lower risk for catching STDs when you are in a mutual sexually exclusive relationship.** This means that you and your partner have sex only with each other. If neither you nor your partner is infected with an STD, then you can safely engage in any sexual activity with each other that you choose.

4. **Learn as much as possible about any new potential sexual partner, but don't accept answers at face value.** Unfortunately, research shows that people lie about things such as how many partners they have had. Researchers suspect people are even more likely to lie about homosexual activity, sex with prostitutes, or the use of illegal drugs.

5. **Avoid high-risk sexual behaviour until you are certain your partner is not infected with an STD.** The most risk behaviours are unprotected anal intercourse and unprotected vaginal intercourse. By "unprotected" we mean engageing in these behaviours without using a condom and a spermicidal containing nonoxynol-9 or *octoxynol.* Also refrain form unprotected oral-genital sex; fisting (insertion of a hand or fist into someone's rectum or vaginal); or rimming (placing your mouth or tongue on or into another person's anus) unless you are certain neither you nor your partner is infected. *Any* activity that exposes a person to blood, semen, vaginal secretions, menstrual blood, urine, faces, or saliva should be considered a high-risk behaviour unless partners are in a mutual sexually exclusive relationship and neither is infected. The AIDS virus (HIV) and other STD organisms can enter the mucous membranes of the mouth, vagina, or rectum and through even

microscopically small breaks anywhere on the skin.

6. Rubbing bodies together without vaginal, anal, or oral contact is also an erotic and a "safer" activity if no semen or vaginal fluids come into contact with mucous membranes or broken areas of skin.

7. Mutual masturbation is both a pleasurable and a "safer" activity as long as semen or vaginal fluids touch only healthy, unbroken skin.

Following are medical conditions or syndromes, which are termed as STDs:

1. **Bacterial vaginosis** means infection of the vagina that does not involve swelling or discomfort. There may be an unpleasant odor, and sometimes a slightly increased vaginal discharge; many women have no symptoms. Causes include infection by *Gardnerella vaginalis* and other bacteria, which have replaced the normal vaginal organisms.

2. **Cystitis** means infection of the bladder and most often affects women. It is relatively rare in men because the longer length or their urethra makes it more difficult for infections organisms to travel to the bladder. Symptoms in women include pain or burning on urination (felt inside the body), frequency and urgency of urination, or blood in the urine. Infectious organisms include *Escherichia* coli and other bacteria found in the gastrointestinal tract, staphylococcus, and herpes simplex virus. Some preventive measures include urinating, even if just a few drops, soon after sexual intercourse and keeping the urine more acidic (which is thought to help kill bacteria) by drinking cranberry juice.

3. **Ectocervicitis** means infection of the outer surface of the cervix. Symptoms can include vaginal discharge and those listed under vaginitis. The following organisms can be involved: herpes simplex virus, Chlamydia trachomatis, Trichomonas vaginalis, Candida albicans, and cytomegalovirus.

4. **Endocervicitis** means infection of the inside of the cervical canal. Symptoms may include vaginal discharge but often there are no symptoms. This is usually diagnosed in the female partner after urethritis symptoms send a male partner to his doctor. Chlamydia trachomatis, Neisseria gonorrhoea, and

herpes simplex virus are the infectious organisms usually involved.

5. **Endometritis** means infection of the lining of the uterus. Symptoms are similar to **PID**: (see below). Infectious organisms include Neisseria gonorrhea, Chlamydia trachomatis, Mycoplasm hominis, Escherichia coli, Gradnerella vaginalis, other bacteria, and perhaps some viruses. With careful testing, several different organisms are often found to be present at the same time.

6. **Epididymitis** means infection of the epididymis. Symptoms may be similar to urethritis or include pain, swelling, and tenderness in the scrotum (almost always on only one side), and fever. This infection can be caused by Chlamydia trachomatis, Neisseria gonorrhoea, and other bacteria.

7. **Infectious prostatitis** means infection of the prostate gland. Symptoms include inflammation (swelling), difficulty in urinating, increased frequency and urgency of urination, pain and burning at urination, following urination. The causes are not very well understood. In some cases STD organisms seem to be involved, but their role is unclear. Men often do not have symptoms for many years.

8. **Nongonococcal urethritis** (NGU) is the term used to describe any inflammation of the urethra (urethritis) *not* caused by gonorrhea. NGU affects both men and women and is one of the most common STDs. NGU is an infection of the urethra caused by bacteria-like organisms. The two most common bacteria involved in NGU are Chlamydia trachomatis in both women and men, and Ureaplasma urealyticum in men. No one is sure how many people are affected. But studies have shown NGU is twice as prevalent as gonorrhea. About 30 percent of infected men have no symptoms. NGU symptoms in men are similar to those for gonorrhea and other urinary-tract infections: a slight discharge from the penis and discomfort while urinating. The majority of women with NGU have no symptoms, although if the organism has also infected the genital tract some report vaginal discharge or pelvic pain. A sore throat can signal that the organism causing NGU is present there, a result of oral-genital sexual activity. Even though NGU can be difficult to diagnose, if it is caused by Chlamydia trachomatis it can be

cleared up in 80 percent of cases by taking the antibiotic drug tetracycline for eight to ten days.

9. **Pelvic Inflammatory Disease (PID)** is a term that is used to describe bacterial infection of the Fallopian tubes, the uterus, and/or the ovaries. Scarring resulting from PID can cause infertility. PID can be caused by Neisseria gonorrhea, Chlamydia trachomatis, other sexually transmitted organisms, and infections related to using an IUD (intrauterine device) and childbirth. PID can also be caused by Escherichia coli; bacteria from the rectum, which may be transferred to the vagina by improper wiping after defecation; or by having vaginal intercourse after anal intercourse without first thoroughly washing the penis. Many women with PID have *no* symptoms, but if symptoms develop they may include tenderness around the abdomen, lower abdominal pain or cramps, cervical discharge, bleeding between menstrual periods, and tenderness when the cervix is touched. In acute PID, a woman may also experience irregular and unusually painful menstruation, pain during intercourse, severe abdominal pain, vomiting, nausea, and headache. Treatment usually involves antibiotics to fight the infection, but some acute or chronic cases also require surgery to remove the infected area.

10. **Proctitis** means infection of the anus and rectum. Symptoms include rectal pain and bleeding, mucous discharge, and diarrhea. This can be caused by STD organisms either as the result of spreading from the genitals (in women) or directly from receptive anal intercourse.

11. **Salpingitis** means infection of the Fallopian tubes. Symptoms are similar to PID and causes include Neisseria gonorrhea, Chlamydia trachomatis, Mycoplasma hominis, Escherichia coli, Gardnerella vaginalis, other bacteria, and perhaps some viruses. Several different organisms are often present at the same time. Salpingitis can also result in infertility.

12. **Urethritis** means infection of the urethra. The name is the same for both men and women. Symptoms in men may include discharge from the urethra, pain, burning and discomfort at urination, and itching at the tip of the penis. Symptoms in women may include urgency to urinate, burning or pain felt inside the body before urine comes out and during urination,

and low abdominal pain. Males are more likely to have symptoms than are females, but many men and even more women have no symptoms. Organisms involved include Neisseria gonorrhoeae, Chlamydia trachomatis, Ureaplasma urealyticum, herpes simplex virus, Candida albicans, Escherichia coli, other bacteria and rarely Trichomonas vaginalis.

13. **Vaginitis** means infection of the vagina that, unlike bacterial vaginosis, does cause swelling and/or discomfort. Symptoms may also include increased vaginal discharge that may have an odor, swelling, itching, burning, or pain in the vagina; and pain with intercourse. Symptoms may worsen during or immediately following menstruation. Organisms involved include Trichomonas vaginalis and Candida albicans.

14. **Vulvitis** means infection of the external female genitals. Symptoms may include burning or pain felt at the urinary opening or on the outside of the genitals after urination begins; increased vaginal discharge; irritation, burning, or itching of the vulva; and sores or lesions on the vulva. Organisms that can cause this include herpes simplex virus, Candida albicans, and possibly human papillomavirus.

15. **Gonorrhea** Neisseria gonorrhoeae is the organism that causes gonorrhea, "clap" and one of the oldest known diseases. Gonorrhea means "flow of seed," probably because the characteristic discharge from the penis was misinterpreted to be semen rather than the symptom of an infection. More than 400 years before the birth of Christ, the ancient Greek physician Hippocrates appeared to have recognized that gonorrhea was sexually transmitted, because he wrote that a disease with similar symptoms resulted from 'the pleasures of Venus." Gonorrhea is almost exclusively transmitted through unprotected sexual activity (or during birth from mother to baby). There is no evidence that transmission occurs from toilet seats or other similar objects. Researchers believe that the risk for woman to become infected by a man is higher, probably because women retain the infected semen in their vaginas.

This organism usually infects the urinary and genital tracts, with the rectum, the throat, and the eyes infected less frequently. Serious illness results if the bacteria spread up the genital tract to infect the Fallopian tubes or epididymis, or if they enter the bloodstream. Infection of the urinary tract is the most common form of gonorrhea in men. Symptoms appear within one to fourteen days, with the majority of men developing symptoms two to five days after infection. The most prominent symptoms are first, difficult or painful urination, followed by the development of a discharge from the urinary opening. Without treatment these symptoms usually disappear after several weeks, and in 95 percent of men within sex months. More serious illness results when the bacteria ascend into the internal reproductive organs and cause infection of the epididymis (epididymitis), the prostate (prostatitis), or the seminal vesicles (seminal vesiculitis). In women, the most common site of infection is the cervix, although 90 percent of these patients will have Neisseria gonorhoeae in the urinary tract as well. Only women who have had hysterectomies are likely to experience urinary-tract infection alone. Infection of the Skene's and Bartholin's glands is also common. A large proportion of women do not develop any symptoms and have what may be called a "Silent" or asymptomatic infection. In those women who do develop gonorrhea symptoms, these are likely to appear within ten days of infection and include increased vaginal discharge, painful or difficult urination, bleeding from the vagina between menstrual periods, and heavy menstrual bleeding. Genital gonorrhea during pregnancy can result in spontaneous abortion, premature delivery, and infection of the amniotic sac (which surrounds and protects the fetus during pregnancy), and infection of the newborn. If untreated, the infection can travel into the female reproductive organs and cause PID. This occurs in about 10 to 20 percent of infected women. Long-term effects resulting from damage particularly to the Fallopian tubes include infertility and ectopic (tubal) pregnancy—a life-threatening situation. Infection of the anus and rectum is involved in 35 to 50 percent of women with infection of the cervix and usually has no symptoms. Forty percent of homosexual men with gonorrhea are infected partner. Men are more likely to have symptoms that include constipation, discomfort or pain, urgency to defecate, bloody stools, and discharge. In a few rare cases, the bacteria invade the bloodstream and cause arthritis and skin diseases.

16. **Syphilis** Syphilis, caused by the organism Treponema pallidum, is a disease whose symptoms can take a vast variety of forms, does not resolve without treatment, can last for many decades in the body. and inevitably leads to death. If diagnosed it can be treated with penicillin and cured. It has great historical importance because of the many influential individuals it affected-from kings to statesmen to artists. Some of its symptoms are described in biblical and other ancient writings. The current medical name comes from a 1530 poem about an infected swineherd named Syphilis. The first European epidemic arose in the late 1400s around the time Columbus returned from America, which led people to believe that the disease had been acquired from the natives in the New World. There is, however, little evidence suggestive of syphilis among early native Americans; other similar disease organisms prevalent in tropical climates may have mutated to become the syphilis bacteria. It is more likely that the return of Columbus and the rapid spread and increase in the severity of syphilis were a coincidence.

Syphilis is most often transmitted by sexual contact. It can be acquired during vaginal intercourse, anal intercourse, or oral sex with an infected partner. Syphilis is usually infectious. However, transmitted from an infected mother to her fetus for many years, although after approximately eight years the risk of maternal/fetal transmission is nearly zero. Unlike gonorrhea, syphilis spreads throughout the body shortly after it enters. If the infection is not treated, it typically goes through three stages. The primary stage is characterized by the appearance of a sore or lesion called a chancre at the site where the bacteria entered the body. The chancre appears between 10 and 90 days after exposure. This is usually a single sore that is rounded, rubbery, and painless. Most often located on the genitals or near the anus, the chancre can also appear on the lips, tongue, tonsils, breasts, or fingers. Even if untreated at this stage, the chancre heals in a few weeks. The secondary stage usually begins within a few weeks or months of the initial infection. It is characterized by a general illness including one or more of the following symptoms: rash, low fever, feeling or general discomfort, sore throat, headache, swollen glands, weight loss, patchy or thinning hair loss, and general aches and pains.

Contact with the rash can result in transmission of syphilis from an infected to a healthy individual. In some cases there are also signs of brain or spinal cord disease; this is called the latency period. The final or tertiary stage is characterized by very serious disability that may involve paralysis, severe psychiatric and mental illness, and then death.

17. **Scabies** The source of the word *scabies* is thought to be the Latin *scabere*, "to scratch". The itch mite was discovered by Bonomo in 1687, and thus scabies was the first disease in humans to have an identified cause. Each mite has four pairs of legs and walks rapidly on human skin until it finds a suitable location to burrow in. This burrow is its home for its thirty-day lifespan. Here the female mite lays eggs for the next generation of mites, which take about ten days to mature. Infested individuals have an average of eleven adult female mites on their skin. Like crabs, the symptoms of scabies are caused by a kind of allergy to the mites: this takes several weeks to develop.

18. **Genital Herpes** This is caused by herpes simplex virus. Despite what might have been led to believe, herpes infection is far from a new disease. The word *herpes* meant "to creep" in ancient Greek and was used in medicine to describe a spreading skin eruption. At the beginning of the second century A.D., the Roman poet Juvenal described sores of the genitals that may have been caused by the herpes virus. Around the same time, the Roman physician Herodotus described the cold sore. In 1736, the physician to the French king Louis XV wrote a description of genital herpes as accurate as any we have today. In 1814 Thomas Bateman, a British physician, described the course of a Herpes outbreak from the prodromal phase to the opening of the sores. Then in 1887 British surgeon Jonathan Hutchinson reported that herpes was likely to recur. Although herpes was understood at the beginning of the twentieth century to be caused by a virus, not until the early 1960s did researchers in Germany and the United States discover there were two types, one most often associated with the face and one with the genitals.

The medical name for genital herpes is herpes simplex virus-2 (HSV-2); the type of herpes that most often causes sores of the mouth and lips is herpes simplex virus-1 (HSV-1). Although each type is most likely to be found in one location or the other, both can infect either site. These and other similar herpes viruses are found in all human populations and, in each, a large number of people are infected.

The first time a person has an outbreak of genital herpes it is called a primary infection. This primary outbreak has the most severe symptoms, including some that affect the rest of the body. Local genital signs can include many painful sores (sometimes in more than one location), itching, painful or burning urination, and a discharge from the vagina or urethra, depending on where the outbreak occurs. Most women also develop an infection of the cervix during their first episode of herpes outbreak.

About 40 percent of men and 70 percent of women also have symptoms that affect the whole body—such as fever, headache, a feeling of general discomfort, and muscles pains. More than half report general symptoms and about one-third have headache, stiff neck, and a mild sensitivity to light. The general body symptoms appear and then disappear within the first eight or nine days. The attack can range in severity from mild to debilitating, but it is believed that many cases are so mild that the individual does not seek medical care. Studies have shown that during the first episode of genital herpes pain lasts an average of nine to thirteen days, and the lesions take an average of fifteen to twenty-three days to heal. Painful sores are reported by 99 percent of women and 95 percent of men. Pain and irritation from the sores gradually increase over the first week and reach their peak between seven and eleven days.

Herpes sores begin as red rounded cone-shaped bumps that develop into groups of small blisters *filled with a clear, very infectious fluid. These blisters then break, leaving a painful opening, and moist sore. If these sores or lesions are not on mucosal tissue they will* develop a crust and then heal. In addition to the genitals, lesions on the buttocks, groin or thighs may also develop (more frequently in women than men) usually in the second week of the disease. These symptoms then decline. In a primary infection, sores are widely spaced and may appear on both sides of the genitals.

After the first outbreak, the virus goes into a state called latency. During this time, the virus is located in nerve cells and in neither active nor infectious. For reasons that are still unclear, the virus becomes active again, causing new outbreaks in the years following the first occurrence. These episodes are called recurrent infections and are characterized by only the local symptoms (sores, pain, etc.) in a milder form and usually appear on only one side. The duration of recurrent outbreaks is briefer: symptoms can vary in severity from one outbreak to another for the same person and are likely to be more severe in women than in men.

About 50 percent of people have symptoms that precede each recurrent outbreak. These feelings are called the prodromal phase and can vary from mild tingling sensations occurring thirty minutes to forty-eight hours before the sores appear at the location to shooting pains in the buttocks, hips, or legs one to five days before the attack. Approximately 90 percent of individuals who have a primary outbreak experience recurrences and about 50 percent of these have five recurrences or more each year during the first two years, with men having slightly more than women. Transmission occurs when an infected area is shedding the virus and comes in close contact with the mucous membranes of another individual (particularly those of the genitalia, mouth, lips, or throat) or small breaks in the skin. Since the virus is easily inactivated at room temperature or by being exposed to air, it is unusual for the disease to be spread by objects like toilet seats or clothing.

Herpes is only infectious and can only be transmitted when the virus is shedding; this occurs mostly from the time bumps appear on the skin to when the sores develop a crust. But to be safe, unprotected sexual activity should not occur during the entire period from the time an infected person first feels the tingling that precedes the eruption of a sore until the lesions are fully healed.

The herpes virus can also be transferred from mother to fetus either during pregnancy or birth. Although initially there was a great deal of concern about transmission during pregnancy and delivery, it has become clear that this is a relatively rare occurrence and caesarean sections are now recommended only for those women who have an active outbreak at the time of delivery. A recent major study indicated that having a *recurrent* episode of herpes during pregnancy had no negative effect on the health or birth weight of the newborn or on the length of the pregnancy. *Primary* herpes infection during pregnancy is a more serious condition resulting in a significantly higher rate of transmission to the fetus. All women who have herpes should seek prenatal care and delivery services from an obstetrician experienced in the management of pregnant women with primary and recurrent herpes.

Diagnosis of herpes is done primarily by physical examination. Use of condoms, *if the sores are fully covered,* herpes prevent transmission of herpes. The addition of a spermicidal containing nonoxynol-9 may enhance protection because this compound has been shown to effectively inactivate herpes virus in the laboratory. Herpes virus can be spread from one part of the body to another, so always carefully wash your hands after touching a sore or putting on medicine. Be particularly careful about touching your eyes after touching a sore or the area around it.

19. Genital warts: These are caused by a virus known as human papilloma virus. In ancient times, warts of the anal and genital (anogenital) area were both well known and common. These warts originally were thought to be a symptom of syphilis or gonorrhea. After the bacterial causes of these STDs were identified, it was then believed that genital warts resulted from irritation or genital secretions. The fact that viruses cause warts was established in the early twentieth century, but until the 1970s it was thought that all warts were caused by one virus. Scientists now know that there are at least sixty types of papillomaviruses, twenty of which can infect the genital tract. Until the middle of this century most scientists did not believe that genitals warts were infectious, but when an outbreak occurred among the wives of American soldiers returning from the Korean war it became clear that indeed they were an STD.

Genital and anal infections with papillomavirus and herpes virus are now considered two of the most common STDs. Genital warts are most common in men and women between 20 and 24 years of age. As with herpes, the number of people infected with human papillomavirus (HPV) who don't have any obvious symptoms is probably much higher than those who are aware that they havc genital warts.

The number of cases of warts on the external genitals is increasing. Because many sufferers never visit a physician for diagnosis and internal warts are not included, these cases represent only a small percentage of the total number of infections. Human Papillomavirus infections are not readily visible.

Anogenital warts come in a variety of shapes and sizes, from so tiny that they cannot be seen even under magnification to very large. Their shape and size probably depend on the type of papillomavirus causing the infection. In men, warts can appear on all parts of the penis, foreskin (if the man is uncircumcised), scrotum, or inside the urethra, where they can cause bleeding and discharge, diminish the flow of urine, or produce no symptoms at all. In women, HPV can be found on the vulva, labia majora or minora, inside the vagina, or on the cervix. Warts around the anus are found in both sexes and have also been discovered in the rectum.

Direct sexual contact between infected and uninfected partners is the most common way in which genital warts are transmitted. In a recent study that investigated the male sexual partners of women diagnosed with genital warts, nearly 70 percent were found to be infected also. As with most STDs, the more partners people have had the more likely they are to be infected. Although HPV was, until recently, considered more of an embarrassment and inconvenience than a threat, several of the types that infect the genital tract have now been associated with precancerous or invasive lesions or tumors of the cervix, vulva, anus, and penis.

As with genital herpes, proper use of a condom can reduce the risk of transmission if all the warts and infected areas are completely covered.

Infection with HPV can be treated and often eliminated. The sexual partners of people diagnosed with this viral infection should always be examined. The earlier treatment begins, the better the result. Before treatment starts, laboratory tests should be done for all other STD organisms that often coexist with HPV. Anyone with genital warts or another form of HPV infection should avoid sexual contact that involves the unprotected affected area until treated and retested to make sure the virus is gone.

Several methods are used to treat HPV and none has been found to be superior to the others. Treatments include painting the warts with substances the destroy them or removing the warts. The best overall treatment strategy is to eliminate all the visible signs of infection and then keep having regular exams to check for any recurrence.

20. HPV-related Cancer. Infection with HPV is associated with genital-tract cancer in men and women, particularly cancer of the cervix. Scientists believe that these viruses stimulate the first step in what is now seen as a *multistep* process that may lead to most genital cancers. One piece of evidence that supports a link between HPV and cervical cancer is the finding that current wives of men whose previous wives had cervical cancer are at increased risk for developing this cancer. The supposition is that these men have carried HPV from the first marriage partner to the second. Once one has been diagnosed with an infection of HPV, one should have regular and frequent *examinations to check for changes in genital tissue.* Remember, cancer diagnosed early can almost always be cured.

21. Acquired Immunodeficiency Syndrome (AIDS). During the 1960s and 1970s physicians noticed cases of individuals whose immune systems appeared to have stopped protecting them against disease. Their immune systems became crippled and infections that usually were easily defeated by the body now attacked with unheard of power, leading to devastating illness and finally death. This condition was not thought of as a separate disease because no one physician saw enough cases to realize that this lack of immunity signaled the existence of an unidentified infectious organism. Acquired Immunity Deficiency Syndrome (AIDS) in the United States and Europe may have been reported as early as 1952 but was not recognized as such.

In the United States it was clear that the outbreak of AIDS was not limited to a few cities or populations; by the end of 1982 over 800 cases had been reported in more than thirty states. Once it was known that AIDS was caused by an infectious organism, the suspicion that it might be sexually transmissible was confirmed when a study of the first 216 cases in southern California found that forty of the men could be linked sexually to one another

What Causes AIDS? By 1984, the disease organism that causes AIDS was identified in France and the United States. After much scientific discussion, the virus was finally named Human Immunodeficiency Virus (HIV). It is a special kind of retrovirus called a *lentivirus*. Retroviruses use the genetic material in the cells they invade to reproduce. *Lenti* means slow; lentiviruses cause infections that take a long time to reveal themselves. This means that months or years may pass between the time the virus invades the body and the time the person has any symptoms of a disease. In the case of HIV, once the virus has entered the body in invades certain cells of the immune system and may reside in these cells for years without any obvious effect; then, in response of some stimulation that it still not clear, the virus uses the genetic material in those cells to reproduce large numbers of itself, destroys and exist the cells, and spreads out to infect many more immune-system cells. Eventually, the immune system and its ability to fight off diseases is disabled or destroyed.

What Does It Mean To Be HIV Seropositive? When a disease organism invades the body, the immune system responds in a number of defensive ways. One response is to develop antibodies against the disease organism; these help the immune system identify and fight the organism. In most cases, the antibodies help cure the disease and then remain to defend quickly against the same disease in the future (this is called immunity). The problem with the AIDS virus (HIV) is that it attacks the cells of the immune system itself, whose job it is to fight and defeat this and other diseases.

Viruses are more difficult to identify as the cause of a particular disease than are bacteria and other organisms because they are so small; therefore the easiest way to find out if a person has been infected with a virus is to test the individual's blood for the presence of antibodies against the virus.

Being HIV seropositive (sero = "blood") means that a person's blood has been tested for the presence of the specific antibodies against HIV (the virus that causes AIDS) and the antibodies were found. When a person is HIV seropositive, we know that the AIDS virus is in the body because the immune system has produced antibodies to it. Scientists also use the term "*seroconversion*" to HIV to mean that the immune system has produced the antibodies associated with a particular disease organism once the organism has entered the body. Seroconversion to HIV infection can begin in as few as five days and be completed by between the second and seventh week after infection. In rare cases seroconversion can take up to a year or more to show up on an HIV antibody test.

Testing for HIV itself rather than for its antibodies is difficult, time-consuming, and expensive. So the vast majority of tests to discover whether a person is infected with HIV are really tests to detect antibodies the immune system has made in an attempt to fight the virus.

What Does It Mean To Have AIDS? Since the AIDS virus (HIV) attacks, disables, and then kills important components of the immune system, the immune system is ultimately unable to destroy the virus. And eventually the virus damages the body's defenses to such an extent that the individual is vulnerable to other disease organisms (opportunistic infections) to which he or she might be exposed; AIDS patients may die from these illnesses even though they don't ordinarily kill.

The course of infection with HIV, which results in AIDS and finally death, is a complex one that is similar in many respects to untreated syphilis—it often starts with some very mild symptoms, disappears for years, and then reappears in a devastating and deadly form.

The majority of individuals first respond to HIV infection with no symptoms at all or with mild symptoms like those for flu or mononucleosis. If mild symptoms do appear, they may include fever, muscle and joint pains, a general feeling of discomfort, tiredness, lack of appetite, nausea, diarrhea, sore throat, or a rash. Headache, stiff neck, eye pains, sensitivity to light, irritability, or depression are also not uncommon. These symptoms may last for two to three weeks and then usually disappear.

After infection, whether the initial period involved symptoms or not, a period of time elapses when the infected individual usually experiences no symptoms. These individuals are called asymptomatic carriers of HIV. In adults, it is now estimated that this asymptomatic carrier state—from infection to the development of AIDS—lasts an average of seven to nine years, although there are healthy-appearing infected individuals who have been symptom-free (asymptomatic) for as long as twelve years. Many individuals with no other symptoms do have swollen glands at several different places in the body; these last for more than three months. This condition, called lymphadenopathy, does not appear to predict when the person will progress to having AIDS—several studies have shown no difference in the timing of the appearance of AIDS between asymptomatic carriers with or without this condition. Although an individual has no symptoms and is likely to look and feel perfectly well, he or she can infect others. Specifically, this means that they can spread the AIDS virus (HIV) to other individuals in the following ways: intimate sexual contact, exposure to their blood, or during pregnancy and delivery of the fetus and during nursing of the newborn.

It is not yet clear what factors are responsible for progression from the symptom-free state to developing AIDS. Such factors as infection with other disease organisms, genetic factors, the virulence of the particular strain of HIV, and life-style (for example, whether or not one smokes or drinks alcohol) have been suggested. After a variable period of being HIV-seropositive, the beginning of AIDS may be signaled by a variety of symptoms, including long-lasting fevers, night sweats, weight loss, diarrhea, and/or the appearance of other illnesses such as shingles or yeast infections.

Following this period, the AIDS patient may experience a great variety of serous problems, which can include any of a number of opportunistic infections, tumors, and nervous system disorders. The AIDS virus has been shown to be capable of directly affecting the skin and mucous membranes, the gastrointestinal tract, the kidneys, heart, lungs, and nervous system. Once a diagnosis of AIDS has been made, most individuals die within two years and few survive longer than three years. The length of survival is dependent on such factors as age, sex, and in what way the disease was acquired.

How Is HIV Transmitted? The AIDS virus (HIV) can only be spread in four ways—through intimate sexual contact, exposure to infected blood or from an infected mother to her fetus during pregnancy or delivery, or to the newborn through breast feeding. Unprotected penile-anal intercourse and penile-vaginal intercourse are the sexual behaviours that have been clearly demonstrated to present the highest risk of sexual transmission. All these activities are only associated with the risk of infection if one of the individuals involved is already infected with HIV. In industrialized nations, it appears that male-to-female transmission is more likely than female-to-male.

Sharing of needles by intravenous drug users is a major route of transmitting HIV not only from one user to another but, secondarily, through intimate sexual activity with their sexual partners.

Although at the beginning of the epidemic many individuals became infected with HIV through contaminated blood transfusions or blood products, now that careful testing of donated blood is routine, that risk has been almost completely eliminated.

After almost a decade of the AIDS epidemic, there is *no* evidence that this disease can be transmitted by casual contact, insect bites, or the handling of food utensils, toilets, and even toothbrushes and razors with an AIDS patient, no cases of transmission have occurred. So the risk of transmission in less intimate circumstances like schools, workplaces, swimming pools, restaurants, and theaters appears to be zero.

How is AIDS Treated? Each seropositive person must find out exactly how to prolong his or her own wellness and how to protect others from infection even though the infected person does not feel sick or have any AIDS symptoms. Keeping well can involve taking better care of your health (including giving up smoking and use of drugs and alcohol, eating a healthy diet, and sleeping enough); taking medicine like AZT (zidovudine), which may prolong health in a *symptomless* HIV-infected person; and practicing safer sex to protect yourself from another exposure to HIV or other STD while at the same time protecting others from your infection.

To date HIV infection and AIDS cannot be cured. However, within three years of the identification of the virus AZT had been developed and was being tested as a treatment. In the original clinical study of AZT in AIDS patients, it appeared to prolong life and reduce the number of opportunistic infections. Till the cure is available of this dreaded disease, the best thing you can do is to avoid infection with HIV (as well as other STDs) by identifing and acknowledging all the factors that may put you at risk and take steps to protect yourself from this deadly virus.

Chapter-9

Sexual Records

"In her abnormalities nature reveals her secrets" – GOETHE

Largest human penis

We all know that men are supposed to worry endlessly about penis size. In popular mythology a small organ is still thought to signal a totally inadequate lover. All the best books tell us that this idea is absurd but nonetheless the notion persists. What can we say of penis size? How big is the biggest? One problem is who is to do the measuring. If men measure their own organs they are likely to exaggerate the results: it is not an area in which there are abundant objective surveys. And women too may exaggerate the size of a particular penis in their acquaintance. Walter (of My Secret Life) demonstrated this clearly enough: a woman spoke of a penis as being 7 inch long or even more – yet the "very large penis" measured by Walter turned out to be significantly less than 7 inch. According to Wardell B. Pomeroy, the Kinsey co-worker, the longest penis encountered was ten inches. The figure accords quite well with the results of the special Forum survey into penis size. In this careful and detailed survey, published in 1970, the largest penis was found to be 9½ inch *in erection, hardly able to compete with the vast organs of pornographic fiction.* In an earlier inter-racial survey, Dr. *Jacobus's* 1935 publication – *"L'Ethnologie du Sens Genitale",* larger dimensions were recorded. In this survey, organs nearly 12 inch in length are reported. Of all penis sizes quoted in the literature the largest is unquestionably the 14 inch erect organ mentioned by Dr. David Reuben in "Everything You Always Wanted to Know About Sex". But as no source is quoted perhaps we should not take too much notice of this figure. The largest well-attested penises would seem to be between ten and twelve inches in the erect state.

SMALLEST HUMAN PENIS

Vast numbers of men – in one estimate the greater majority – think that they have a penis much below the average in size. Perhaps they should console themselves with the thought that many men have extremely diminutive organs. Pomeroy states that the smallest penis encountered in the Kinsey surveys was 1 inch long. In the *Forum* study the smallest erect penis was found to be 4.75in. in length, quite large compared with many of the specimens that do exist. There are instances reported in the medical literature of penises that do not exceed 1 cm. in full erection: such organs are sometimes labeled with the appropriate term *"micropenis"*. And even 1 cm. is not the smallest-sized penis known to medical researchers. There is a condition known as congenital *hypoplasia*, where the body of the penis is totally absent and the glans is attached to the pubic region. In one such reported case, with an effective penis of much less than 1 cm. in length, the testes and secondary sexual characteristics were found to be quite normal.

LARGEST PENIS BY RACE

In the Dr. Jacobus survey definite penis size differences on a basis of race were detected. The largest Arab penises were found to be between eight and ten inches; but it was among the Muslim Sudanese that Jacobus found "the most developed phallus" – notably "one of the maximum dimensions, being nearly 12 inch in length, by a diameter of 2¼ inch" The hardy researcher remarked that this was "a terrific machine" – "more likely the penis of a donkey than of a man". He concluded that the "Sudanese Negro possesses the largest genital organ of all the races of mankind". In a less extensive survey, but equally interesting, Dr. Robert Chartham measured erect penises for groups of men of various nationalities. The largest organs for each nationality were as follows: English – 10½ inch; West German 8½ inch; Negro – 7½ inch; French – 7¾ inch; Danish – 8 inch; American – 7¾ inch; and Swedish – 7¾ inch The groups were small, ranging from only 9 to 121 individuals; nevertheless the data acquired are not without significance.

SMALLEST PENIS BY RACE

In the Jacobus survey the Hindu man was reckoned to have a penis that only averaged around 4 inches, a much smaller figure than for the other races investigated. In the Chartham survey the smallest organs in the various nationality groups were as follows: English – 2¾ inch; West German – 3½ inch; Negro – 4 inch; French 3½ inch; Danish – 5 inch; American 3½ inch; and Swedish – 5 inch. As we have already suggested, with the groups being rather small no racial conclusions can be drawn.

LARGEST HUMAN TESTICLE

Testicles are much of *muchness,* varying in dimensions very little from man to man. One authority, T.H. Van de Velde in his "Ideal Marriage", puts the "mature testicle" at from 4 to 4½ cm. long, and from 2 to 2 4/5 cm. broad. It is suggested that "at the utmost" the testicle does not exceed 5 cm. in length. This is probably true for healthy men, though venereal and another diseases can produce staggering results. In some maladies a testicle the size of a football is not unknown. One can only try to imagine the agony caused by elephantiasis and other conditions in which the testicles can swell to proportions vastly larger than the victim's head.

HEAVIEST HUMAN BREASTS

Massive breasts, as we all know, fascinate many men. Magazines cater specifically for such tastes and a number of striptease artists try hard to *capitalise* on gigantic mammary apparatus. In one recorded instance ("The Sexual Anatomy of Woman" by W. F. Benedict), a girl of fourteen had breasts weighing sixteen pounds; and in another case a woman of thirty had breasts weighing fifty-two pounds. As with the male sexual organs breasts are sometimes grossly enlarged by disease or some other unwelcome cause. For instance some women have hypertrophied breasts, sagging vastly and of quite giant proportions.

MOST PENDULOUS BREASTS BY RACE

Breasts come in all shapes and sizes and hues. We have already noted some massive specimens: there are other ways in which breasts can be excessively dimensioned. They can, for instance, be extremely long, dangling like strips of skin. This occurs in a number of African tribes and can be common in both young and old women. It is not unknown for women to toss their breasts over their shoulders to keep them out of the way while working.

LEAST PENDULOUS BREASTS BY RACE

The smallest and leait pendulous breasts are usually attributed to the Mongoloids. Among such people the women often appear with an almost boyish slimness – and the vast *mammaries favoured* in other parts of the world would be regarded as monstrous deformities.

LONGEST HUMAN CLITORIS

Clitoris size has only rarely been of importance in human society. A few communities – Ford and Beach mention the Easter Islanders – have favoured the large clitoris and some natives have tried with varying degrees of success to enlarge this organ in their girls. For the most part, however, with a prevailing indifference in the nineteenth-century and early part of the twentieth-century to sexual arousal in women, the clitoris has been neglected. Needless to say, it varies in size. How big are the largest? Theo Lang in "The Difference Between a Man and a Woman" mentions one recorded instance of a woman having a clitoris 2 inch long, and 3 inch "When fully erect". Pomeroy has remarked that clitoris measuring more than 1 inch are very rare in whites, but may occur in 2 or 3 inch and more were obtained from perhaps one out of 300 or 400 black women". Benjamin and Masters note in "The Prostitute in Society" that parent-*Duchalet* came across a woman with a monstrous clitoris no less than 7 inch long. But the record clitoris is almost certainly the 12 inch specimen mentioned by various writes and quoted (without comment) by W. Francis Benedict in "The Sexual Anatomy of Women".

LONGEST FEMALE PUBIC HAIR

Pubic hair, short and curly in most of us, sometimes grows to quite extraordinary lengths. Havelock Ellis worked as a midwife in his early days, and he notes that only in one case did long pubic hair hamper his efforts. In some remarkable cases recorded by a certain Mr. F.L. John (1778-1852) the pubic hair was longer than the women's ordinary hair. Thus *(Paulini):*

the pubic hair reached the knees.

EARLIEST GROWTH OF MALE PUBIC HAIR

Pubic hair, normally a sign on the onset of puberty, can occur – as can menstruation –at a surprisingly early age. H. Jolly mentions a boy of only eighteen months who had both an enlarged penis and pubic hair. Often such conditions are associated with a number of other abnormalities. In the cited case the boy "presented with a right-sided abdominal mass." Autopsy showed the mass to be a primary *hepatoblastoma.*

LARGEST GROWTH OF FEMALE PUBIC HAIR

In some women there is a little pubic hair growth at any time. Such a circumstance can occur in women sexually normal in every other respect. In yet other women pubic hair may eventually grow in a completely normal way but may commence growth at a surprisingly early to late age. In the Kinsey survey some women did not have any pubic hair until they reached the age of eighteen. It is unlikely that this is a record. We may reasonably speculate that some women in their early twenties have not yet started to grow hair in the genital area.

EARLIEST GROWTH OF FEMALE PUBIC HAIR

In Kinsey report, some girls began growing pubic hair as early as eight years of age. This is very young to begin such growth yet cannot be considered "abnormal." Hugh Jolly noted instances of pubic hair in babies, in one case a girl of only one month old had hair growth around the genitals.

OLDEST WOMAN TO MENSTRUATE

The onset and termination of menstruation is subject, like all other phenomena, to immense variation. It has been known for a girl to start menstruating at three months old (H. Jolly in "Sexual Precocity", Proc. Royal Soc. Med. 44, 1951), and occasionally the menopause too occurs at a very early age: there are instances of girls reaching the menopause before the age of twenty. The menopause rarely occurs after the age of fifty-five but rare cases do occur. In one instance menstruation was continuing in a woman aged 104.

LATEST TO MENSTRUATE

Menstruation, commonly functioning in the vast bulk of teenage girls, may be delayed well past the teens. In a number of cases medical attention needs to be sought; in others the condition may exist in a "normal" but "slow" girl. In the Kinsey sample some girls did not start menstruating until they were in their twenties. The latest instance was a girl who started to menstruate when she was twenty-five years old.

FIRST DISCOVERY OF SPERM

Human sperm were first discovered by a student of Antonij van Leeuwenhoek in 1677 in the city of Delft. The name of the student is not known for certain: he is variously written up as Ludwig Hamm, van Hamm or von *Hammen*. According to some writers he is a Dutchman, to others a German. One day he brought to the acknowledged master of microscopy, Leeuwenhoek, a bottle containing semen and pointed out the small animals could be seen moving about in the ejaculate. Van Leeuwenhoek went on to study the seminal emission from a wide range of sick and healthy men; in the semen of them all the odd creatures could be detected. He described his findings to the Royal Society in London .

"I have seen so excessively great a quantity of living animalcules that I am much astonished by it. I can say without exaggeration that in a bit of matter no longer than a grain of sand more than fifty thousand animalcules were present, whose shape I can compare with nought better than with our river eel. These animalcules move about with uncommon vigour and in some places clustered so thickly together that they formed a single dark mass. After a short time they separated. In fine, these animals astonished my eye more than aught I had seen before".

Of course at the end of the seventeenth-century there was still a mystery as to what sperm actually were. Some thought them to be parasites in the seminal fluid – and saliva and urine and other bodily secretions were quickly examined in the search for more sperm. Others thought them coagulating agents.

FIRST DISCOVERY OF SPERM AS FERTILIZING AGENT

It was not realized that sperm were concerned in the process of fertilization until the nineteenth century. Various names are associated with the discovery – Prevost and Dumas (1824), Peltier (1835), and Dujardin (1837).

FIRST SPERM BANK

The idea of an effective sperm bank has appealed to eugenically minded individuals for a good few centuries. Such arrangements have only recently become practically feasible. The first two sperm banks, set up in Lowa City and Tokyo, *both began life in 1964.*

FIRST SPERM-BANK CHILD

The first sperm-bank child was born in the U.S. in 1953 – and, in the words of Gerald Leach, was "perfectly normal". Since then the numbers have swelled, with the sperm storage period being gradually lengthened.

MOST FAMOUS VICTIMS OF VD

A great number of famous and talented men have had one sort of venereal illness or another. They are Caesar, Charlemagne, Henry VIII, Richelieu, Casanova, Boswell, Goethe, Keats, Nietzsche, Mussolini, Hitler, Oscar Wilde, etc. This list could easily be extended.

MOST EXTREME REACTION TO CONTACT WITH SEMEN

Most women don't mind semen too much, though some unduly fastidious ones complain about its smell or stickiness. Some females, however, have a quite extraordinary reaction to seminal fluid: they are happily rare. In one case reported in 1967 a girl had an acute allergic reaction to human sperm. She came from a family with a long history of various kinds of allergy, including eczema, asthma, and dermatitis. A short time after her first sexual experience she developed a rash and asthma; her lips, eyelids, tongue, and throat became swollen, she had violent pains in the pelvis and finally lost consciousness. Most of these symptoms appeared every time she had sexual intercourse: they began within half an hour and lasted well into the next day. When semen diluted one part per million was injected under her skin it left an angry weal, so intense was the girl's reaction.

OLDEST APHRODISIAC

Some aphrodisiacs have been popular since the days of antiquity. The mandrake plant is mentioned in the Old Testament and is still in use today. Mandrake (or *madragora, mandragora officinarum*) is a member of the potato family with a large dark-brown root and small red fruit. It contains the alkaloids atropine and scopolamine: in mild doses these are soporifics; in large doses they can kill ! In antiquity there were magical rules for harvesting the plant. Pliny noted that the plant roots were in the form of human genitals – which explains, through the idea of sympathetic magic, the supposed aphrodisiac effect. Cantharides, another ancient aphrodisiac, was first mentioned by Aristotle: its active principle, *cantharidin*, is extracted from the dried and powdered bodies of the blister beetle, a brown or bluish creature found in southern Europe. Yet another old alleged aphrodisiac is ginseng, the "mystic plant of the Orient", made into tablets by modern sex aid retailers and also into a wine. In the Far East today ginseng wine is *termed kaoling* (as strong as vodka), with the roots of ginseng soaked in the cask for at least three years. Users are recommended to take a small glass before going to bed.

MOST FAMOUS ORIENTAL APHRODISIAC

Despite the legendary nature of ginseng most in the West are more likely to have heard of the various uses to which opium has been put. This drug has in fact been employed optimistically as an aphrodisiac over the centuries. Even a mild dose of opium is supposed by Orientals to provide about one hour of continuous genital stimulation – "assuring the desideratum of at least three thousand phallic thrusts".

LEAST SENSITIVE EROGENOUS ZONE

Many men are keen to play with a woman's vulva: women are often relatively indifferent to such activity – particularly if the man focuses on the outer lips. The inside lips (labia minora) are usually highly sensitive; the outer lips (labia majora) much less so. The women surveyed by Fisher rated the sexual excitement areas in the following sequence clitoris, vagina, near clitoris, inside lips of vulva, inside vagina, and breasts. The outside lips of the vulva were rated the least excitable of all.

OLDEST POTENT COUPLE

All relevant surveys have shown men and women still having sexual intercourse when in their eighties or even nineties, though around three –quarters of all men are impotent by the time they reach their eighties. The oldest potent male in the

Kinsey survey was an 88-year-old Negro, who continued to enjoy regular sexual intercourse with his ninety-year-old wife! It should be said that some cases of impotence in old men are certainly due to the absence of adequate stimulation: though it is arguable that sudden stimulation to orgasm in an old man could prove fatal as has happened.

LONGEST MAINTAINED ERECTION

For some purposes it may be desirable to maintain an erection for a long time. It is clear that periods of up to an hour are not uncommon, and that if the penis is in the vagina for this time then maintaining an erection is not difficult for some individuals. Kinsey noted that the length of time over which the erection can be maintained under "continuous erotic arousal" drops from an average of nearly an hour in the late teens and early twenties to seven minutes in men in their late sixties. It is pointed out that under prolonged stimulation "many a teenage male will maintain a continuous erection for several hours . . ."

FASTEST ERECTION

Speed of erection varies enormously from one man to another – and in the same man from one sexual encounter to another. Factors such as alcohol and fatigue are highly relevant, as is the degree of erotic arousal. In a few exceptional males the erection of the penis may occur in as little as three seconds.

OLDEST INDIAN SEX MANUAL

The oldest and best-known Indian sex manual is the "Kama Sutra of Vatsyayana", written about 1500 years ago. It has been pointed out that this comprehensive volume summarized many earlier writings on sexual topics dating back as much as three thousand years. The first English edition of the "Kama Sutra" was privately printed in 1883; the Indian "Ananga-Ranga" was translated into English ten years before the "Kama Sutra". This latter, more important work is the first full manual from India devoted exclusively to the subject of human sexuality and in particular to the relationships between the sexes.

MOST FAMOUS EROTIC SCULPTURE

The most famous erotic sculpture in the world is certainly that of the Hindu temples of India. Most of the best examples were created in the North between the ninth and thirteen centuries A.D., and in the South between the sixth and seventeenth centuries A.D. The sculptures show every imaginable form of sexual activity – different coital positions, oral sex, masturbation, rape, bestiality, etc. The carvings, elaborate and meticulously executed, show all forms of sexual behaviour.

Chapter-10

Sex after Forty

The epoch-making work of William H. Masters and Virginia E. Johnson has become the most famous sex research since that done by Kinsey and his colleagues. Their book, *Human Sexual Response,* which described what happened to people during intercourse as observed under laboratory conditions, rose spectacularly on the best-seller lists almost immediately after publication and remained there for many months.

A major contribution of their research—but one less known to most people—is their work on the response of older persons.

A number of other investigators have surveyed the sexual behaviour of older persons. Masters and Johnson were the first actually to investigate the anatomy and physiology of sexual response in person over forty.

In this part of the study they had sixty-one menopausal and postmenopausal women (ages forty to seventy-eight) and thirty-nine men (ages fifty-one to eighty-nine). Obviously, these numbers were not large enough to provide complete statistical data and further studies will be required. But they furnished important preliminary information.

When the orgasmic cycles of the women of this group were studied, Masters and Johnson found that generally the intensity of response to sexual stimulation was reduced with advancing years through all phases of the sexual cycle. Specifically, the sex flush was more limited and restricted in the older women, there was less lubrication; there was delay in reaction of the clitoris to direct stimulation, and reduction of duration in orgasm time. However, they emphasized, they did find "significant sexual capacity and effective sexual performance" in these older women.

There seems to be no physiologic reason, they concluded,

why the frequency of sexual expression found satisfactory for the younger woman should not be carried over into the years after the menopause, with no time limit drawn by the advancing years to mark the end of sex activity.

As in the female, Masters and Johnson found that as men get older the intensity and duration of physical responses during the orgasmic cycle were reduced. Particularly after sixty, erection takes much longer, ejaculation lacks the same force and duration, and the sex flush in markedly reduced. "There is no question," said Masters and Johnson, "that the human male's sexual responsiveness wanes as he ages."

However, they added, with regularity of sexual expression maintained and with a sexually stimulative climate within the marriage, a healthy male's capacity for sexual expression could extend beyond the seventies and the 80-year age level.

One of the points that Masters and Johnson keep emphasizing in their discussion of the factors necessary for maintaining sexual capacity and effective sexual performance is regularity of sexual intercourse. This, they say is essential for both men and women.

For example, in the later years, thinning of the vaginal walls and reduced lubrication make intercourse uncomfortable and often painful for the woman. However, in three women past sixty years of age the vagina was repeatedly observed to expand and lubricate effectively despite obvious senile thinning of the vaginal walls and shrinking of the outer lips. These women had maintained regular intercourse once or twice a week for their entire adult lives.

On the other hand, women in the stage of five to ten years after the end of menstruation who had intercourse infrequently (one a month or less) and who did not masturbated with regularity had difficulty in accommodating the penis during their rare exposures to intercourse.

Regularity of sexual expression is also the key to sexual responsiveness for the ageing male, say Masters and Johnson. With loss of sexual outlet, many ageing males report rapid loss of sexual tension and potency.

One of the problems faced by women in their postmenopausal years is the loss of estrogen brought about as the ovaries reduced their production of hormones.

Masters and Johnson note that, as the women moves through her postmenopausal years, the lining of the vagina becomes very thin. Instead of having the thick, ridged pattern characteristic of the vagina when it is receiving considerable estrogen stimulation, the walls of the vagina become tissue-paper thin; therefore, they cannot protect the structures lying next to the vagina—the urethra and bladder-by absorbing the mechanical irritation of active intercourse. There is also a shortening of both vaginal length and width and a shrinking of the outer lips, leading to narrowing of the opening of the vagina.

In addition, once the woman is about five years past the menopause, the rate and amount of lubrication production diminish to an obvious degree. This is not true for all women, since Masters and Johnson observed three women over sixty, who consistently responded to sexual stimulation with rapid production of lubrication typical of women under thirty. All three of these women had very active sex lives throughout their mature years.

Another result of hormone imbalance is that contractions of the uterus, which take place during orgasm at all ages, now become painful. For some women these contractions are so painful that they seek to avoid orgasm and even intercourse itself.

As a result of these changes, intercourse during the post-menopausal years may be difficult in many ways. Some women find penetration and the friction of intercourse painful. Some complain of a burning on urination, which develops from mechanical irritation of the urethra and bladder because of the thrusting movement of the penis. It is not unusual for many to have an urgent need to urinate immediately after intercourse.

Fortunately, today it is easily possible to make up for any lack of hormone production in the body with adequate hormone replacement therapy. In some cases, local application of a simple lubrication between the lips of the vulva will relieve the discomfort entirely.

If the tissues are very thin and tender, estrogen creams or suppositories applied locally to the vulva and vagina may restore the tissues to normal layers and cure the discomfort within a week or two. In addition, more and more women are being given general replacement therapy to make up for the loss of hormone production by the ovaries.

At any rate, masters and Johnson point out; the effect of hormone imbalance after the menopause on sexual adjustment is not completely established. Sexual performance in many cases depends far more on opportunity for regular intercourse and on numerous emotional factors than it does on hormone imbalance.

In their clinical work with older males (as distinct from the laboratory research), Masters and Johnson found six general categories of factors which were responsible for loss of sexual responsiveness during the later years: (1) monotony of a repetitious sexual relationship (usually translated into boredom with the wife); (2) preoccupation with career or economic pursuits; (3) mental or physical fatigue; (4) over indulgence in food or drink; (5) physical and mental infirmities of either the man or his wife; and (6) the "fear of failure."

Many others besides Masters and Johnson have noted the problem of monotony, which is probably the single most important factor in the loss of an ageing male's sexual interest and responsiveness. Kinsey and his colleagues described it as "psychologic fatigue" the fact that there is just not as much psychological stimulation in an experience that is repeated without too much novelty or variation with the same partner over an extended period of time.

Of course, it would be wrong to place all the responsibility for weakening sexual response on the wife. In many cases, Masters and Johnson reported, men were so preoccupied with their careers that their outside interests were all-consuming, becoming a major deterrent to sexual activity in the home, particularly when communication between husband and wife was poor.

Excessive consumption of either food or drink also has a tendency to repress sexual feelings, and Masters and Johnson found that secondary impotence developing in the late forties or early fifties has a greater connection with excessive drinking than with any other single factor.

It is clear that, as men age, they have an increasing number of minor, or in some cases major, physical disabilities, each of which may in some way lower sexual responsiveness; where the wife is affected, it may restrict opportunities for sexual intercourse for the husband, often putting an end to sexual life altogether.

Although as has been noted, these researchers found important physiological changes in sex responses occurring as the years go on, their major conclusions are sharp and clear: "There is no time limit drawn by the advancing years to female sexuality" and under proper physical and emotional conditions for the male there is "a capacity for sexual performance that frequently may extend to and beyond the 80-year-age level."

Chapter-11

Overcoming Premature Ejaculation

"I come so soon that Priya doesn't have time to reach her own orgasm. What's wrong with me? What should I do?" Rahul, the young man speaking, had been married less than a year when he and his wife, Priya, consulted a sex therapist. At that first meeting, they expressed great disappointment and frustration with the sexual aspect of their relationship. Rahul was depressed.

"I'm really turned on by Priya," he said. "Maybe that's part of the problem. I'm so stimulated that I climax within a minute or two after penetration."

Rahul's problem is widely referred to as "premature ejaculation" – a fancy name for a remarkably common difficulty. Almost 50 per cent of all men in sex therapy sought it because they feel they ejaculate too quickly. Although the condition is most prevalent among men in their late teens and 20's, it also occurs in older men. The typical premature ejaculator is a man like Rahul: physically healthy, with a high sex drive, and no difficulty achieving erection. The problem is entirely one of ejaculatory control. Fortunately, men who fit in this description can almost always be helped by the newer sex therapy techniques.

What is premature ejaculation?

The definition of premature ejaculation varies, depending very much on who is doing the defining. For example, a wife may feel that her husband ejaculates too quickly if he climaxes before she's reached orgasm—regardless of the actual amount of time spent in intercourse. By this definition, a man who can engage in sexual thrusting for 15 minutes might still be called "premature" by a woman who needs 30 minutes to reach orgasm.

In the past, many men considered rapid ejaculation to be a sign of health and masculinity. Nowadays, a man is more likely to be concerned with his partner's sexual satisfaction. So, while a quick ejaculation may not be a problem for the man, he knows that it is often a problem for his partner, and he's likely to try to "hold off" until she reaches orgasm. When he can't, he feels that he has a sexual problem—that his ejaculation is "premature."

How do sex therapists define "premature ejaculation?" Most of them want a definition that takes into account the satisfaction of both partners. For example, Masters and Johnson feel that the man who reaches orgasm before his wife at least 50 percent of the time is a premature ejaculator.

Other definitions focus on the man's ability to control his ejaculatory response. In her book 'The New Sex Therapy', Dr. Helen Kaplan states that "prematurity is a condition wherein a man is unable to exert voluntary control over his ejaculatory reflex, with the result that once he is sexually aroused, he reaches orgasm very quickly." According to her definition, the time spent in intercourse is far less important than a man's ability to control ejaculation.

How fast does the average man reach orgasm? In 1948, Kinsey reported "for perhaps three-quarters of all males, orgasm is reached within two minutes after the initiation of the sexual relation." He also found that many men regularly climax within 10 or 20 seconds of penetration, and that ejaculation even before intercourse begins, was not uncommon. Since 1948, other research has confirmed that, for a majority of men, ejaculation occurs within five minutes of penetration. In my opinion, if a man ejaculates before 80 or 90 active coital movements or thrusts should consider oneself suffering from premature ejaculation.

Some *"common sense" remedies for premature ejaculation:*

A quick glance through almost any popular men's magazine indicates not only how widespread the problem is, but also the large number of "cures." A man is invited to choose from a variety of special lotions or ointments that diminish, or numb, sensations in the penis. Condoms are often recommended for the same purpose.

Another popular technique is distraction. The premature ejaculator is advised to concentrate of nonsexual fantasies to keep himself from being aroused past the point of no return.

The theory is that, in thinking about the stock market, or mentally reviewing the batting averages of his favorite ballplayers, he will be able to hold off until his partner has had her orgasm. Physical distraction—tensing his anal muscles, for example during intercourse—is also recommended.

In addition, locker room folklore has it that strenuous exercise, a cold shower, or masturbating just before lovemaking will lower the sex drive and thus delay the ejaculation.

According to Dr. Kaplan, "common sense" remedies are rarely successful. With them, intense arousal might indeed be somewhat delayed or diminished, but it is not likely that the ejaculation itself will be slowed.

Aside from that, there is a very real drawback involved: Since the purpose of the "common sense" remedies mentioned above is to lessen sexual arousal, they also tend to lessen the pleasure of lovemaking—and pleasure is the very thing we want most in sex.

The role of anxiety: A man who thinks he ejaculates too quickly is likely to be anxious about it. A vicious cycle develops. For example, the more anxious Rahul was, the faster he ejaculated—which only made him even more anxious the next time around—and so on. When he was most anxious about his performance, he'd avoid making love entirely. Naturally, when he finally did try intercourse again, after a period of abstinence, he would ejaculate even more quickly.

Masters and Johnson have suggested that, for some men, may be related to stressful conditions during a man's first sexual experiences. Furtive lovemaking in the backseat of a car, for example, is hardly conducive to relaxed and controlled orgasms. Unfortunately, a pattern of rapid ejaculation may develop and persist long after the pressure to complete the sex action quickly has been removed.

Other sex researchers, Dr. Wardell Pomeroy among them, believe that anxiety is the basic problem of the man who ejaculates very soon after penetration. Pomeroy speculates that, at high levels of sexual excitement some men experience intense anxiety, which triggers a premature orgasm.

The squeeze technique:

Rahul and Priya's problem was typical of many that have been treated successfully by sex therapy. The most common choice of treatment is the squeeze technique. A form of this treatment was first developed in 1956 by Dr. James Semans. Later, it was modified by Masters and Johnson, but the principles are still the same. A success rate of over 90 per cent has been reported for couples who carefully follow the instructions given by their therapist.

Usually, when the squeeze technique is employed, the wife is instructed to stimulate her husband's penis with her hand. At the moment of inevitability—the point when the husband feels he is about to have an orgasm—he signals her. She immediately—and firmly—squeezes his penis between her thumb and forefinger. A firm squeeze will not hurt the penis, but it will stop the orgasm.

After several practice sessions with manual stimulation, the couple resumes intercourse. The female-superior position is used. The wife is instructed to remove—and firmly squeeze—her husband's penis when he signals that he is near orgasm. Three to six weeks of conscientious practice is usually enough to make a big difference in the couple's sex life.

The squeeze technique enables the premature ejaculator to lower his orgasm threshold. With his partner, he learns to experience intense sexual excitement without having an immediate orgasm. He gains greater control over his need to ejaculate, and learns to climax when he chooses to.

A new treatment for early ejaculation:

At their first meeting with the therapist, Rahul asked if his sexual behaviour was normal. The answer was "yes." Though premature ejaculation can lead to sexual incompatibility between a husband and wife, it is rarely a sign of biological abnormality. The male of other species, such as chimpanzees, usually ejaculate within 20 seconds of entering their mates. According to Kinsey, the human male who ejaculates quickly has an intense response, which is actually a sign of good health and normality.

The therapist who saw Rahul and Priya believed that in their cases rapid ejaculation was not at all surprising, considering how young they were and how quickly they turned on by each other. The "problem," in fact, arose from the way they reacted. Instead of trying to slow Rahul's response, the therapist chose an alternate method of working with the couple: teaching them sexual options and encourageing them to view their sexual relationship in new ways.

First he asked about their typical lovemaking sessions. "It always begins with petting. Then Rahul gets an erection pretty fast," Priya explained, "and we begin intercourse. While we're making love I keep thinking that soon it will be all over. Within a couple of minutes, Rahul has a climax. Then, we both feel disappointed and frustrated because we know that's the end. Rahul loses his erection and is very angry with himself. I'm upset because I haven't had an orgasm. That's how we're feeling as we fall asleep.'

The therapist explained that theirs was a very common reaction to quick ejaculation, but that there are other ways to view the situation. For example, he said, instead of seeing Rahul's ejaculation as a problem, Priya could interpret it as a sign that he is enormously turned on by her. His quick ejaculation is a compliment.

He explained that the difficulty, if there was one, was that both Rahul and Priya saw his ejaculation as the end of their lovemaking. But it could also be seen as the beginning. As a young, healthy, sexually active man, there was no reason to assume that one Rahul had an orgasm, he had to fall asleep. After the first orgasm, he could instead relax and concentrate on giving Priya sexual pleasure.

It's true that a man is likely to lose his erection after he ejaculates. He enters what is called the refractory period—an indefinite time, which must pass before he is able to attain another erection. It varies between man and man and is not necessarily constant even for a particular man. But that need not mean the end of a lovemaking session. There is no reason why he cannot continue to give his wife pleasure. He can stimulate her manually or orally in ways that he knows will excite her to orgasm. It's important for him to realize that an erection is not necessary for him to be a good and effective lover.

For her aspart, the wife needs to stop thinking of intercourse as the only she can experience sexual fulfillment; there are many other different, but satisfying ways. She should be clear and assertive about the kinds of stimulation she likes. In that respect, the more she expects from her husband, the more she's likely to receive. He wants to be an effective lover and her orgasm is proof of his success.

Rahul and Priya followed their therapist's instructions and were pleasantly surprised at the results. They continued lovemaking after Rahul's ejaculation, and he found that he could easily be aroused a second time. Frequently, he regained a firm erection and was able to resume intercourse. Priya learned to experience sexual pleasure and orgasm in a variety of ways. Their sex life was expanded to include many new and exciting ways of enjoying each other.

At their final therapy session, Priya described the changes in their lovemaking. "Rahul and I wanted our sex life to be fulfilling for both of us. We thought that his premature ejaculation was a problem keeping us form that goal. I can see now that what we did together in bed was restricted. We both came to this marriage with very little sexual experience, and not much imagination about our sexual options.

"Now we know that good sex doesn't depend on an erect penis. Even if Rahul ejaculates immediately, we can go on with our lovemaking. We experiment. We aren't stuck in a single pattern. We're both more relaxed, because we know that Rahul's ejaculation is only the beginning. And a lot of the time, he lasts much longer now."

No one would have thought that Rohit had any serious problems to look at him—he was good-looking, intelligent, getting ahead in his profession although still in his mid-20s—and women invariably found him attractive. But his relationship with the opposite sex never continued after first few dates, despite his wit and charm. His male friends thought of him as a real swinger, never suspecting the truth: After a minute or two of lovemaking, Rohit climaxed, and it was all over for him and his partner. Sometimes he would wait a while and try again—with the same result.

Prakash – a divorced man in his early 30s—was even more unlucky. Since he'd started seeing women again, he invariably had an orgasm before he could enter his partner's vagina. Try as he might, he was unable to delay this early response.

Both Rohit and Prakash suffered from the most common sexual disorder known to Indians: premature ejaculation. More important, they soon realized that their difficulty was not an occasional, but a persistent one; and when that became clear, they lost no time in seeking help. Millions of other men who suffer from this difficulty are too embarrassed to admit that what is wrong. Yet, there are many methods of overcoming it, some of them discovered rather recently. Of all male sexual disorders not related to disease, premature ejaculation is actually the simplest to deal with; in most cases, it can be easily and quickly overcome.

Most sexologists agree that not every man who cannot hold his own orgasm back until his partner has her climax is a premature ejaculator. (Some women require as much as an hour of stimulation before they can attain orgasm. In such cases it is a female, rather than a male sexual difficulty, which needs treatment.) But if a man can't hold back long enough to satisfy the average, properly aroused woman – say for at least five minutes or a bit longer—it's likely that he is the one with the problem.

Premature ejaculation is not only a cause of sexual incompatibility but also of resulting general emotional distress. The premature ejaculator frequently has feelings of inadequacy in other, seemingly unrelated, areas. It's important for him to realize how widespread his difficulty is. About half of the men in this country have suffered from the same problem at one time or another.

Sex clinics and related institutions throughout the country have recently initiated programs to deal with this condition. The procedures outlined in the present article are based on the findings and recommendations of many sex therapists and researchers and may be tried by the average man afflicted with the problem of climaxing too early. As long as he has no physical disorder related to his ejaculation difficulty, the odds are that the following procedures will help him to overcome the condition permanently.

1. Start and stop technique: This Technique was originated by sexologist James Semans. That is the most basic of all the new methods of ejaculation control, because it is the simplest and most direct example of the desired result – to stop the oncoming orgasms at will. It is the easiest to practice and takes the least preparation. Ideally, it should be tried first alone, and later on with a sexual partner.

After you have made yourself as comfortable as possible in a situation where you are sure not to be disturbed, arouse yourself physically as you would ordinarily do before masturbating. Provide yourself with anything that will turn you on erotically – a drink, music, soft lights, pictures, comfortable pillows and cushions, and so on.

Then start manipulating your penis and other parts of your body until you get an erection, and continue until you feel that you will have an orgasm soon. Up until that point do not hold back, but put as much vigor into the act necessary to enjoy the experience thoroughly.

At the point you feel ejaculation approaching, however, cease all movements and other activities that would otherwise lead to climax—and wait. Just wait, until the urge to climax subsides. That should happen in less than a minute. Then, slowly, proceed to masturbate again; continue as before, and stop at the same point as you did previously. That is the stop-start exercise; repeat it three to six times before you allow yourself the release to ejaculation.

For maximum effect, the exercise should be done on the average of once a day for approximately two weeks. At first you may reach orgasm earlier than you intended; that is normal, however, so don't get discouraged. After a few days you will know much more about your personal reactions and timing and be able to control your sexual responses more fully. After a week or so, the stopping periods may be decreased in time to only a few seconds, and the actual number of these "stops" can be increased to 10 or more in a given session before you reach a well-deserved orgasm.

After two weeks or so of this technique and the consequent buildup of orgasmic control, your next step should be to try traditional sexual intercourse with an understanding partner. (Ideally, she should be someone with whom you have had sex before. She would not only be more likely to be understanding, but you would also be in a better position to anticipate her responses. She'd be less likely to do something unexpected that might bring on an early climax).

Continue using the stop-start method; by now, it should scarcely be noticeable to your sexual partner, since the pauses, as mentioned above, will be brief. If necessary, withdraw from vaginal penetration partly or completely for a few seconds if you feel that otherwise you will reach the point of orgasmic inevitability. After a while, you will probably find even that unnecessary and you would be able to delay your ejaculation for much longer time than before.

2. The Squeeze technique: This technique is also evolved by Semans but made famous by Masters and Johnson. Also called Masters and Johnson's technique. Having treated 168 men by this technique, suffering from premature ejaculation at their sex clinic in St. Louis (U.S.A.), the noted team of Masters and Johnson report, they had only 4 failures. Another famous sex therapist, Dr. Helen S. Kaplan of the Cornell University Medical College, points out that the success rate is both very high and usually permanent. This technique attains ejaculation control that can be practiced in privacy at home. Again, masturbate just as you would for the sheer enjoyment of it; but, when you feel that you may ejaculate soon, grasp your penis slightly beneath its head and hold it tightly for about 20 seconds or so—until the urge to climax subsides and your erection loses some of its firmness. Rest shortly in that position, and then repeat the process once more. That should be done about three or four times during each "session."

After a few times, you should be able to gauge how soon to squeeze how hard, and at precisely what spot to apply the pressure for maximum effectiveness. The underside is usually the most effective spot on which to concentrate.

(Bear in mind, however, that squeezing the penis head itself will probably bring on the ejaculation rather than retard it. Also, once you have passed the point of orgasmic inevitability it is useless—and often harmful – to try the procedure. So don't squeeze when you feel that it's too late. Just squeeze earlier the next time.)

Once you have mastered the technique by yourself, it can be tried during lovemaking with a partner, during intercourse or any other form of lovemaking. Within two or three weeks you should show a marked increase in ability – to hold off climax until you – and she – are good and ready for it.

3. General Experimentation: When Amita and Ajai both realized that he definitely suffered from premature ejaculation, they decided that, rather than focus on one specific technique for overcoming it, they would try different methods, often simultaneously. They'd stick with the ones that seemed to work best, until the problem was overcome.

First they tried to "take off the pressure," which was recommended by Ajai's doctor. Rather than indulge in regular lovemaking that always ended in intercourse, they petted and engaged in other forms of love play for a few nights.

"It was like extended foreplay," Amita stated later. "Ajai had no fear that his penis would be over stimulated to the point of ejaculation, and I climaxed often without any difficulty, even though we weren't actually having intercourse. That built up his ego tremendously."

Within a week they were having intercourse again, but Ajai was extra careful in every respect: he went very slowly at first, withdrawing completely whenever he felt that he was nearing the point of ejaculation, still maintaining nonpenile contact with his girl. At first he used a condom, even though Amita was on the Pill, to minimize sensation in the penis and prolong the sex act. Later, he used an ointment, which gave extra lubrication and desensitized his penis, although he reported that in two or three nights he no longer found such artificial aids necessary.

Other methods they tried included Ajai's emptying his mind of erotic thoughts as much as possible when he felt climax approaching too rapidly, achieving orgasm by other means (such as masturbation) an hour or two before intercourse, and during intercourse shifting to a circular movement instead of the usual thrusts.

For her part, Amita reported that whenever she felt that Ajai was approaching climax before she was able to do the same, she would hold him off – sometimes asking or motioning him to stop his thrusting or actually withdraw for two or three minutes – meanwhile making sure that the lovemaking continued, although actual intercourse had been modified or interrupted. She also encouraged him to stimulate her genital area in other ways, thus bringing herself to climax sooner in addition to delaying Ajai's.

According to the final report, since Ajai and Amita were open and free with each other, rather than embarrassed and guilt-ridden, their problem was almost completely solved in less than a month, without the help of any special books, techniques, or sex specialists.

4. Different Positions in Intercourse: Although the man-on-top woman-beneath position is the most common and satisfying to many couples, it can bring on the male orgasm very fast. When the female is on top, straddling the male, she can receive equally strong stimulation without comparable stimulation of the penis, as the pressure comes in a different area. The side-by-side position often has the same effect, since the man is then able more easily to move freely in more directions, thus stimulating his partner without penetrating too deeply and running the risk of ejaculating before he wishes to. Penetration from behind, with the woman's posterior slightly raised, while her weight is mainly on her arms, is a third position which affords her keen sensations while keeping the chances of a man's climaxing to a minimum. Moreover, in all of these variations, it is easier for the man to use his hands and fingers in manipulating the woman's clitoris. In many instance she may climax more than once before more standard intercourse is resumed, and the man finally has his own orgasm.

5. Change - of – Pace: One of the most common – and natural – methods of prolonging a sexual interlude is to switch from straight intercourse to another equally satisfying mode of sex for brief periods before ejaculating. After five minutes or so of vaginal penetration, for instance, one might "take a break" from that from of sexual activity and give her oral sex. That will not only give your penis a rest period, and allow your approach to orgasm to subside, but it may also afford both you and your partner a variety in your sex life that many couples have never experienced.

During that "intercourse intermission" sex will not stop; in all probability, you will maintain your erection throughout, but without danger of achieving orgasm too early.

6. Specialized Professional Help: If none of the above techniques seem to bring results you consider satisfactory – if they help very little or not at all – that doesn't mean that the problem is insoluble. Within the last decade, sex therapy clinics under medical supervision have sprung up in every area of the country. In addition, there are many private sexologist and psychotherapists who specialize solely in matters such as these. It may be difficult at first to overtly admit to yourself that such help is needed, but, if after trying some or all of the methods described in this article you feel that advice and treatment by an accredited specialist is indicated, there is no good reason to avoid seeking such help.

In any case, as crucial as the problem of premature ejaculation is in one's sex life, it can be treated successfully in just about every instance, because of the increase in knowledge and technology available in the last few years.

Chapter-12

Physical causes of Impotence

- Diabetes
- Obesity
- Excessive Weight Loss
- Use of Drugs
- Organic Nervous Diseases
- Organic Injury

This article deals with impotence caused by some organic, local or constitutional disorder—that is, physical impotence—as distinct from purely functional impotence caused by emotional problems. Generally speaking, sexual potency depends upon 4 things: sex drive, erection, ejaculation and orgasm. These 4 factors, however, are not equally concerned as causes of impotence. The successful completion of the sex act on the part of the male depends mainly upon effective erection. This is the basis of male potency, and without it the normal sex act is impossible. The other factors are not necessary for the satisfaction of the man's female sex-partner. Male impotence is often a result of some physical disorder of the sexual apparatus, which may include inherited or acquired malformations of the male sex organs, or inflammations and degenerative changes affecting the sex organs. A well-known British urologist, says: "There can be no doubt that in such cases there is a lesion (sore or wound) somewhere, which we are perhaps not advanced enough to detect, but the fact that it is hidden does not warrant us to assume that there is nothing wrong." A New York urologist, in a study of 300 cases of impotence, reported that 44 per cent of the patients gave a history of gonorrhea, generally involving the prostate gland and the seminal vesicles.

Eighty-five percent of these had some lesions in the urinary tract. As a result of these tiny sores, it is believed that the sexual nerve centers in the lower spine and the brain are being bombarded constantly by impulses from these parts. The result is irritability or exhaustion of the sexual center, and eventually impotence. It is well known that there are many diseases that are accompanied by sexual difficulties. Sexual problems, including impotence, are especially prone to occur in diabetes. Indeed, very often impotence is the first complaint that brings the patient to a physician and leads to the diagnosis of this disease. One English textbook on diabetes states that about half of the patients troubled with diabetes complain of impotence.

Another condition often accompanied by sexual problems is obesity. There seems to be a connection between an increase in bodily weight and a decrease in sexual virility. The cause of this is not quite clear. It should be noted, however, that the opposite, a loss of bodily weight, is not generally accompanied by a corresponding increase of sexual potency. It is known that excessive loss of weight in weakening diseases, malnutrition or starvation, as, for instance, in prisoners of war or inmates of concentration camps, is often accompanied by a loss of sexual vigor. One exception to this is the tuberculosis patient, who often shows an increase in sex drive and potency, even in the advanced stages of the disease. Certain drugs, when used in excess, are known to affect sexual potency. Camphor, belladonna and arsenic, for instance, are sexual depressants. I once saw patient with psoriasis, a common chronic skin disease, who as a result of prolonged treatment with arsenic, developed impotence, which disappeared when he stopped taking the drug.

Alcohol, morphine, cocaine and nicotine are definitely anaphrodisiacs—that is, sexual depressants. When used to excess, they diminish sexual potency. It is interesting that at the beginning of these drug addictions there often occurs an increase of libido and potency, but prolonged and excessive use is invariably accompanied by a partial or complete loss of sexual powers. Chronic alcoholism usually results in delayed ejaculation. It is believed that the excessive use of nicotine contributes to the development of impotence. This has been demonstrated in numerous animal experiments. Many nervous diseases are associated with sex difficulty or loss of sexual function. In the last stages of syphilis, loss of potency may be one of the earliest symptoms. In some other nervous diseases, especially those associated with injuries of the spinal cord, there may be partial or total loss of sexual potency, depending on the location of such injuries. Sex drive, however, in these cases is usually preserved or even may be increased. With all men, and with some earlier than others, impotence begins, as the man grows older. Normally, in the ageing man, sexual potency subsides gradually with a simultaneous decrease of sex drive.

There are, however, enormous individual differences in the decrease in sexual abilities and not the years alone but the whole make-up of the individual is of prime importance. Frequently we see comparatively young men who are sexually weak while some old men are vigorous in every respect. The sex life, in my observation, goes sooner in those who were never virile and disappears latest in those who were more vigorous. Where there are physical or mechanical obstacles to the sex act, the treatment should be surgical. Prostatic massage, whirlpool and heat treatments, when properly applied, may prove very beneficial, if only for their psychological effect. When impotence is associated wit some internal disease, obesity etc., treatment of the underlying disease should be given.

Chapter-13

Is Bigger Really Better ?

One noticeable result of the present continuing trend toward the tearing down of sex taboos is that males of all ages are concerned with the physical size of their reproductive organs. Many, in fact, are complaining quite openly of an apparent "reduction in size" of their most cherished symbol of manhood. Others are afraid – quite unnecessarily according to all authorities – that when the opportunity presents itself for indulgence in sexual intercourse, their equipment will prove inadequate.

Such complaints stem from the fact that far greater emphasis is being given these days to *sex capacity* in both the male and female. In many cases both sexes now hold the mistaken impression that length, width, and great expansion are invaluable physical assets when it comes to making full and satisfying use of the male sex organ. The root cause of such serious misconceptions is that old devil – 'prudery'. In spite of the recent advances toward sexual emancipation, prudery regarding the external genitalia of the male is still ingrained in our way of life. In thousands of medical articles and papers published in scientific journals every year, very few experts make reference to the penis or the scrotum. Yet women's magazines you can buy openly on the news-stands have for many years, felt completely free to recite and explain the most intimate details of the female sexual anatomy. This full and frank treatment is commendable, but apparently it is not considered proper to mention the sex organs of the other half of the population. Every day physicians are being asked the same worried questions concerning penis size, and the relation of both to sexual intercourse. Here are a few of the questions being repeated over and over again in doctors' offices:

- "When flaccid, my penis shrinks to about 1 ½ inches. This is embarrassing when I am in the presence of other men, and gives me a very uncomfortable feeling. Would taking sex hormones make my penis protrude more? When erect, my penis is five inches long."
- "When having sexual intercourse is it necessary for the male organ to extend the full length of the woman's vagina in order for her to reach full satisfaction? In other words, if the man's penis is too small in relation on the woman, is it possible to satisfy her?"
- "Does the length of penis a woman can accept depend upon the amount of sexual experience she has had? What would happen if she were forced to accept too large an organ?
- "All my buddies seem to regard any man with less than a five-inch organ as a 'shorty,' incapable of giving a woman as much pleasure as those males equipped with larger organs. As a result I find myself obsessed with the desire for a giant sexual organ. Is this normal – and possible?"
- "I have noticed that men with king-sized sex organs are admired and envied by other men. Is their sex performance any better than that of men possessing average size organs? And do women, too, prefer large ones?"
- "Does physical size, height and weight have any influence on the length and thickness of the male organ? Can anything be done to lengthen the organ and obtain a much longer erection?"
- "I am 21 years old and have never had sexual relations. My penis and testes are smaller than normal and I have always thought that sexual intercourse caused these organs to grow to normal size. However, I recently was told that this is not true. Since I will soon be married, I would like to know if I can expect to have a larger penis after regular intercourse. Mine is five and a half inches when erect."
- "What is the normal adult penis size?"

This last question is the essence of the sex problem worrying most virile men. Here is the straight, true answer with no frills or euphemisms, as given by many authorities.

The erect male penis can range in length from just a little under four inches to about eight inches, and from less than an inch to over two inches in diameter. From a statistical point of view this is the normal range, so that the "average" penis is six inches in length and about one and two-fifths inches in diameter.

There are a few men whose sex organs exceed or fall short of the four-to-eight-inch limits. Folklore describing human penises of enormous size are just that – folklore, meaning fanciful lies. In the non-erect or flaccid state, the human penis can vary very widely in size. But at erection these variations between different men usually even out, with the result being the most men tend to fall into the range quoted above. A man with a small flaccid penis will often, at erection, equal in size a man with a larger flaccid penis. The female vagina is by no means as deep as imagined by some men, who feel that they are less than men if they do not occupy it fully. Measured from the hymen or proper entrance, the average depth of the vagina is only about three inches. Repeat: three inches. To this may be added the length of the vulva outside the entrance, bringing the combined average vaginal length to from 5¼ inches to 5¾ inches.

The average erect male organ of six inches can, therefore, easily occupy the full length of the vaginal canal. Furthermore, if the organ is thin and the vagina wide, or if it is short and the vagina deep, appropriate changes of position during sexual intercourse can easily adapt the organs to each other. Actually, the vagina is an elastic tube, resilient and strong, and its walls are well able to adapt themselves to the size of the male organ unless the latter is quite abnormally small – which would be very unusual. In addition, the indisputable fact is that the female clitoris – the area of very great erotic sensitivity – is located outside the vaginal passage and its stimulation does not require a very large male organ. The "reduction in size" complained of by many males is a myth. Once adulthood is attained the true size of the penis is both flaccid and erect states remains constant. The impression of shrinkage is due simply to the fact that an incomplete erection may have taken place. Even when sexual excitement seems adequate, worries, fears and preoccupations may decrease the influx of blood to the organ and thus prevent complete erection. It is significant that those men who feel sexually inadequate are the chief complainers of a reduction in size. Even in aged men there is no real reduction in size, but only a slowing down of the blood circulation and lessening of the sexual desire. The remedy: much stronger preliminary stimulation, which can be most successfully applied by the female partner.

Another significant factor about size complaints is that in cold weather or during a cold bath, the male organ may seem frighteningly small. The man becomes worried and is easily led into thinking that it is actually becoming smaller, which it certainly is not. Cold merely causes a momentary contraction.

Nothing can be done to increase penis size in a normal adult. No administration of hormones or anything of the kind will bring about any change. Penis size, like other organ sizes, is determined by heredity. At puberty the penis begins to grow from its childish dimensions to full adult size including size at erection. After physical maturity has been reached, the penis has reached its final growth. Like penis size, vaginal size is also determined by heredity at puberty. But as we have seen, the vagina is really so elastic and accommodating that we cannot speak of its size in the same specific way.

The importance of penis size to a woman's sexual satisfaction is assessed as "negligible" by most marriage and sex experts. This is because most of the sexually sensitive nerve endings of the vagina are found in the outer third of this organ, near the vaginal opening. The inner two-thirds of the vagina has fewer nerve endings and therefore experiences much less sexual sensation, if any. Females are singularly less concerned about small penis size than are men. Many doctors have never come across a single instance in which small penis size has seemed to be a factor in poor adjustment, except in the imagination or belief of the male concerned. One male patient, possessing the smallest penis his physician had ever seen, married a woman with the largest vagina the doctor had ever encountered. Yet they both told him that their mutual enjoyment of intercourse was of extremely high quality. The amount of sexual experience a woman has had would not have much influence upon the length of the penis she could accommodate. Most women can accommodate practically any penis since, as already explained, the tissue of the vagina stretches to such a great extent. If, by some remote chance, too large a penis were inserted, pain would be felt and the woman would not willingly permit complete insertion. One research team in Sweden interviewed more than a thousand wives whose husband had organs measuring from three to four inches when erect. All these women had experienced intercourse with men of normal dimensions either before or after marriage.

The result of these interviews showed that while some of the wives complained about certain aspects of their husband's performance in the marriage bed, not one of them had found their husbands deficient because he was a "Shorty." A considerable number of them wrote flippantly: "It isn't what a man has got – it's how he uses it."

The myth that sexual intercourse will increase the size of the penis ought to be squashed, too. It will increase in size from the flaccid to the erect state, but not permanently. A penis that is five inches long will serve perfectly satisfactorily as a copulative organ since the clitoris and vaginal entrance – the most sensitive areas of a woman – require practically no penetration for stimulation. Nor will masturbation causes an increase or decrease in size of the male organ. The belief that an increase will occur is based on the fact that boys generally discover masturbation at the time when their sexual organs begin a period of very rapid growth. This is why some begin to think there is a definite connection between the two. The belief that masturbation will result in a decrease in size stems from unfounded guilt on the part of the masturbator. His sexual upbringing has wrongly taught him that such a sex practice is wicked and that shrinkage of his organs will be the outcome. This is utter nonsense. One unlikely theory that seeks to explain the male craving for bigger-than-average sex organs is that such craving is instinctive. It dates back to the time, centuries ago, when men were undoubtedly blessed with larger organs than we have today.

The theory stresses that the penis is, first and foremost, an organ to make easy the introduction of male sperm into the women's vaginal canal. Thus, the longer the penis, the further inside the sperm would be ejected and the greater the chances of pregnancy. This was supposed to have been a biological necessity when Man started out with the apes millions of years ago. At that time Homo Sapiens had to reproduce to their fullest capacity or face extinction. The reasons for this were twofold. In the first place women seldom bear more than one child at a time – as opposed to dogs or cats, say, who bear up to six offspring in each litter. Secondly, the pregnancy period of nine months was much longer than in any of the other species evolving at that time. According to the theory, man compensated for these limitations by assuring himself of impregnation by a foolproof method of copulation involving the long penis. But Man was so successful as an evolutionary experiment that his continued existence on the planet was more than assured in terms of numbers. There was no longer any need for such a high pregnancy probability – the world was already becoming overcrowded by humans by the year 1600. The urge to copulate, however, is an inherited response that no amount of conditioning will ever be able to erase, and therefore some lesser change, on the physiological level, began to happen instead. This was the development of a shorter penis in the male throughout the human race. It did not, however, completely erase the instinctive desire of the male to possess nature's original concept of an efficient sexual organ – a long one.

Whether or not this theory has any basis in fact, (apes have relatively small penises), men still worry about their penis size because there is a deep-seated belief in all of us that well-endowment is symbolic of masculine virility and a greater power to impregnate the opposite sex. Those who are beset by doubts concerning the length of their organ should realize that such doubts are baseless. With proper knowledge of preliminary lovemaking, even a much smaller than average penis should in no way interfere with attainment of complete satisfaction for both sex partners.

Chapter-14

Woman: The Stronger Sex

Men's manners are not they were since women acquired the vote and full equality with men, some forty years ago. Yet we still continue to call women members of the *weaker* sex. There are of course fields of sports such as the boxing ring, in which men display greater strength then women do. But is the boxing ring a satisfactory yardstick with which to measure strength? Personally I am of the opinion that the term the "weaker sex" is a term which should now be scrapped. During a trip to Kenya, some fifty years ago, I watched Kikuyu women carrying loads which were far heavier than the loads which my own safari porters were carrying, and Kenya is not the only country in which women work as hard, if not harder, than men do. But it is in the struggle for survival, rather than in the field of physical work, that the female sex displays its toughness. A slightly larger number of boys are born than girls every year, the ratio in most white races being anything between 101 and 108 boys to every 100 girls. But if we include stillbirths and miscarriages in our statistics, the preponderance of males over females increases. It would probably be true to say that approximately 150 boys are conceived to every 100 girls.

Nature appears to have made this provision in order to compensate for the fact that, constitutionally speaking, males are less resistant to injury and disease than are females. Not only is the greater susceptibility of the male to accidents shown by the greater number of male deaths in the womb; there is also a higher mortality rate amongst males throughout the whole of life. Insurance statistics also show very clearly that wives usually outlive their husbands. In June 1950 there were 6,771,000 people or retirement age living in Great Britain, and of these 4,506,000 were women. o also are women who live to the age of 100 much more common than men who do so.

What is the explanation of this greater longevity of women? Formerly it was suggested that men were shorter-lived because they were frequently engaged in unhealthy or dangerous occupations, such as coal mining. But this explanation is no longer tenable, because women are now engaged in many of the more dangerous and unhealthy jobs that were formerly performed only by men. Even in the industrially advanced countries this is so. Women drive vehicles, work in factories, and in some countries do heavy construction work. They also run risks from which men are entirely exempt, such as the risks of childbirth. And it is in this dangerous occupation of childbearing that we find the explanation, which accounts for woman's greater longevity. Nature has endowed her with special reserves of strength in order that she may carry out her major function, the perpetuation of the race. This is no light task. The heart of a pregnant women has to supply, not only the needs to her own body, but also those of the developing child. Her lungs must provide additional oxygen to the blood, her metabolism must be intensely active, and every organ has to work at a higher pitch. All this is usually managed successfully, thanks to the fact that woman has been given special reserves of energy. But, at a certain age, nature relieves her of this great responsibility of the perpetuation of the race. Then she is free to use her reserves of strength solely for her own purposes. And so she uses them to combat the degenerative changes of old age.

It is not suggested that this is the sole reason for women with-standing the ravages of time better than men do. Woman is better equipped for old age, psychologically as well as physically. I have been struck by the rapidity with which many men, previously busy and fully occupied, have declined after retirement from what has hitherto been their greatest interest in life, their own business or profession. This has been particularly noticeable when these men have never cultivated any hobby or interest outside of their business or profession. But women are much less likely to find themselves deprived suddenly of all motives for living. A woman is a specialist in "personal relationships" and this is an interest she need never give up.

In fact, a woman never retires at all from life and there is no reason for her to become bored, or to lose all zest for living. Consequently she is much better equipped, psychologically, for old age, than her husband is, and she usually manages to outlive him. It is for these reasons that I regard her as belonging to the *stronger* and not to the weaker of the two sexes.

Chapter-15

The Hormone — Testosterone
That Makes you A Man

A man's testicles perform two major functions that affirm and contribute to his biological maleness. They produce and store the sperm cell that is ejaculated in his seminal fluid when he reaches orgasm – and they contain a special cluster of cells that produce a remarkable male sex hormone, known as testosterone. There are a number of other male sex hormones, but testosterone is the most well known. Thought a relatively few researchers question its reputed functions, most agree that it works in both wondrous and unexpected ways. Testosterone causes young boys to mature sexually. Yet, over time, it can change due to ageing, drugs, and medications, even shifts in mood. In many ways, therefore, some well known and some not, it has a profound effect on a man's sexual functioning, and his "maleness." (Women produce very small quantities of testosterone, and it also seems necessary for their sexual functioning – but it's of overriding importance to men.)

The growing body: Testosterone is in the human body from birth, but in minimal quantities and without acting in significant ways. That changes dramatically when a boy reaches puberty. At puberty the pituitary gland goes to work and "orders" the testicles to produce testosterone (as well as other sex hormones) in large quantities. Those hormones then pour into the blood stream and shoot out to various parts of the body. The result? The boy's sexual organs grow in size. His "wet dreams" and spontaneous erections, erections over which he has no control, begin. His voice deepens, his shoulders broaden, his muscles harden, and the beginnings of a beard appear on his face. In the main, testosterone is the sex hormone responsible.

Checks and Balances: Throughout a man's life, his testicles constantly manufacture his all-important testosterone, keeping him sexually capable and active. Amazingly, though, the quantity produced is always very small. Testosterone is so powerful that the tiniest amount suffices to bring about all those marvelous effects. Minute as the output is, if it's less than normal the male is in trouble. Sexual interest wanes or disappears altogether. Effeminate traits may develop in him. Adolescent boys whose testicles don't manufacture enough testosterone suffer from retarded development of the sex organs. At best it takes them much longer than usual to mature sexually. Does that mean every male ought to wish for an overproduction of testosterone – that the more his body makes the more virile and sexually active he'll be? Things don't work out that nicely. In the growing boy, excessive amounts of testosterone may just mean precocious development–that he becomes physically mature much sooner than the other boys do. But adults who overproduce testosterone sometimes show excessive (uncontrollable) sexual drive and exaggerated masculine characteristics, which can be very troublesome.

Highs and lows: A number of researchers have tried to find out whether testosterone goes into the blood stream at the same steady rate all day long. Apparently it doesn't. Some studies show a biological rhythm to testosterone secretion: the highest levels show up in the blood at eight to nine in the morning, followed by a sharp decline from nine to noon. That is probably why many men prefer sex in the morning. Testosterone levels may also be higher during sexual activity. For an unusual study, published in the Journal of Endocrinology, a married volunteer was examined. For 45 consecutive days, his wife, a registered nurse, took blood samples from him once in the morning, once during sexual relations but before he reached orgasm, and once within five minutes after he climaxed. Researchers analyzed the testosterone levels in all those blood samples; they found that the man's testosterone levels were much higher during and right after sex than they were when he wasn't having sex.

Impotence and testosterone: Adult men who become impotent often jump to the conclusion that there's something physically wrong with them – that maybe they're not producing enough sex hormones. But things are generally not that simple.

Roughly 90 percent of all impotence problems are thought to be emotional in origin, rather than resulting from physiological causes. On the other hand, it's true that certain physical ailments can lower testosterone levels or in other ways produce impotence. Physical problems that often result in impaired sexual functioning range from diabetes to multiple sclerosis to tumors. Mumps in grown men is believed to reduce testosterone levels, sometimes causing impotence. Certain tumors will lower the hormone levels, as will certain thyroid disorders and such ailments as Cushing's disease, a pituitary disorder. Recent medical research shows that emotional stress and depression, too, can markedly lower testosterone levels. A tough day at the office or a transitory blue mood aren't likely to do it – but chronic, consistent stress or depression will cause those changes. As soon as the stress is overcome or the depression lifts, testosterone level quickly goes back to it's normal state. Dr. Helen S. Kaplan, who heads the Sex Therapy and Education Program at the Payne Whitney Clinic of New York Hospital, is one of a number of sexologists who feel that every impotent male ought to have a complete medical checkup. Such checkups should include tests for diabetes and other impotence-producing illnesses, and should include a determination of the level of testosterone in the patient's blood. Unfortunately, tests to determine testosterone levels aren't routinely done; in fact, they're expensive and not always available.

How medications affect testosterone levels: Not only certain illnesses, but also a number of over-the-counter medications affect testosterone levels adversely. Researchers have only scratched the surface in this area, but some things are known. It's known that most of the medicines used to lower blood pressure tend to produce impotence in quite a few men who take them, though in this instance factors other than lowered testosterone levels play a major part. Men on estrogen (female hormone) therapy following operations for cancer of the prostate can count on lowered sex drive and lowered testosterone levels; estrogen counters the potency of testosterone. (It's something that, unfortunately, they must learn to accept; reducing testosterone levels in such instances helps reduce the risk of cancerous cell erupting again). The pain killer codeine, if taken for any great length of time, reduces testosterone levels. The commonly prescribed "mild" tranquilizers like Librium and Valium are apt to cause a decrease in sexual performance if taken in large quantities over a period of time; whether they directly affect the production of testosterone isn't clear. Some drugs used in the treatment of allergies, drugs like cortisone and ACTH can counter the stimulating action of the male sex hormones.

Testosterone therapy: Testosterone is more than a sex hormone produced in the body; it's a medication, too, in the sense that it's commercially available and can be injected into the body or taken orally in tablet form under a doctor's supervision. Some clinicians believe that men whose sex drive is low or who show low levels of testosterone can be helped by being put on testosterone replacement therapy. Other clinicians believe that testosterone, whether injected or taken orally, has no more effect than a sugar pill – that patients who improve do so because they've been told they will; that It's all mental. The fact remains that some middle-aged and older men who feel a waning of their sexual powers – and become markedly depressed as a result – report renewed vigor plus a new feeling of well-being when put on testosterone therapy. (Because a lift in spirits is so commonly reported by men undergoing testosterone therapy, researchers at the Worcester State Hospital in Massachusetts are now experimenting with it as a possible treatment for depression itself). On the other hand, it's fair to state that a lot of men who go through testosterone replacement therapy don't feel any improvement at all. At present the most honest thing that can be said about testosterone therapy is that it helps some men but is certainly no sure cure. Men who have cancer of the prostate, or who are suspected of having it, are never given testosterone treatments. And there are a number of doctors who refuse to administer it to any male patient, under any conditions. They feel there's always a danger that the treatment might activate dormant cancer cells. Of course, there are may other doctors who feel that this approach is unnecessarily conservative. Oddly, testosterone treatments help some women, too. Mainly, these are women who have undergone certain kinds of ovarian and adrenal operations, as a result of which they lose all sexual desire. Testosterone therapy sometimes restores their ability to become aroused and enjoy sex.

Drug use and testosterone: Though heavy alcohol use impairs sexual functioning, there's no evidence that it specifically lowers testosterone levels. That's not the case with some other drugs, even those that have acquired a reputation for enhancing sexual performance. Marijuana is an important case in point. Many pot smokers insist that marijuana makes them feel sexier and that they enjoy the sex act under its influence much more than they would otherwise. But at the famed Reproductive Biology Research Foundation in St. Louis, Drs. Robert Kolodny and William H. Masters have found that the levels of testosterone among pot-smokers is an average of 44 percent lower than among non-smoking men. Marijuana smokers who smoked the most had the lowest levels of all. When three of the subjects gave up smoking pot for two weeks, their testosterone levels shot back up to normal. Another testosterone study was done with methadone, the drug widely used to treat heroin addicts. he researchers, from Washington University School of Medicine in St. Louis, found that methadone sharply lowers testosterone levels. In fact, three-fourths of the numerous methadone patient studied said their sexual performance was nowhere as good as it had been before they began the methadone treatment.

How ageing affects a man's testosterone levels: Starting in their late 40s or early 50s, a majority of men experience slightly diminishing testosterone levels. But the change is really nothing to worry about. As Dr. Helmut J. Ruebsaat points out in *The Male Climacteric*, "for 85 percent of men the hormonal change is hardly noticeable". The rest do suffer from a "rapid premature ageing of the testicles," he says, and the result is a "rapid decline" in the amount of male sex hormones their bodies manufacture. But it should be stressed that such men are well in the minority. And as men grow still older? Some evidence shows that androgen (another male sex hormone) output declines steadily but very slowly until a man reaches the age of 60 or so. From then on it remains fairly constant, some clinicians believe. As less sex hormones are produced, though, the man's sex drive and sex activity do diminish – but they don't have to stop.

Happily, researchers at the Duke University's Center of the Study of Ageing have discovered that there's no age limit beyond which men stop having sex. Even men in there 80s and 90s are still manufacturing testosterone – and, at least in some cases, contentedly enjoying its effect.

Chapter-16

Anxiety and Sex

All of us are prone to worry about something throughout our lives. When this worry causes a high degree of mental tension, it is termed anxiety. If the anxiety excites a considerable amount of mental stress, it causes and prevents the normal functioning of the brain and other organs of the body.

It is important to distinguish between what may be termed realistic anxiety and irrational anxiety, the latter being what the psychiatrists term anxiety neurosis; in other words, an emotional or mental disorder accompanied by obsessional anxiety.

To define the two types of anxiety—*realistic* anxiety is the mental apprehension one feels when faced with certain situations whose outcomes we cannot foresee, e.g. taking up a new job, sitting for an examination on which one's future career depends, and even marriage. This type of anxiety is short-lived. As soon as we realize that the new job is within our capacity; as soon as we are confronted by the examination paper to whose questions we know the answers; as soon as we have had experience of marriage and find that it is a desirable life-situation and that we can cope with the domestic and sexual adjustments it demands; our anxiety disappears. Being the kind of creatures we are, we were justified in being anxious about how we would face up to the new specific situation, and since we are predominantly rational beings, as soon as the threat of the unknown has vanished, our anxiety disappears.

Irrational anxiety is quite different, for by definition it exists when there is no obvious or apparent danger. No amount of persuasion that there is no need for worry will convince, or, indeed, that if there is any cause for worry the situation does not warrant the degree of worry evinced. People who suffer from this type of anxiety often develop peptic ulcers, and others develop colitis (inflammation of the large intestine) or asthma, while extreme forms can bring about heart disease.

These physical complaints obviously require medical treatment, but this on its own rarely brings about more than an alleviation of the condition. It should be accompanied by psychotherapy, which will rid the mind of the mental origins of the neurosis.

I mentioned at the beginning that worries could inflict themselves on us at all periods of our lives. Even children are susceptible to mild attacks of irrational anxiety. They worry about their misdeeds (which they inflate), they worry lest they lose the love and affection of their parents, they worry about a subject they are studying with, to them, not very great success, even though they are not doing so badly when compared with their classmates and the teacher has made no adverse comment on their work.

Fortunately, these irrational anxiety states are short-lived, but they may produce, while they are operative, bed-wetting, chronic headaches, nightmares, acute stomach aches, diarrhoea or vomiting. Once the child is reassured that his/her worries are groundless, which pre-supposes that the cause of the anxiety is discovered, the physical disorders and the mental worries can be quickly dispelled.

At the other end of the scale is the late-middle-aged man or woman who worries about his/her continuing ability to function sexually as he/she enters later life. Unfortunately, such cases are all too frequent. Their worry begins when the sexual functioning is more than adequate. Within a short period, however, he/she is dysfunctioning sexually.

Because the mind has such a powerful influence over physical sexual functioning, the tension and mental – and consequent physical – fatigue caused inevitably by the anxiety, makes the sexual organs practically always the first of the organs to be affected. On the other hand, irrational anxiety about sexual dysfunction, *which occurs at all ages,* is one of the commonest causes of actual sexual dysfunction.

Among my current patients is a young man of 22. Since he was fifteen he has suffered from an anxiety neurosis that he will never be able to father children. As a result, he suffers from retarded ejaculation. I got his semen checked and found vigorous sperms but did not allow him to see the report. On the first occasion, I told him that though his semen contained active sperm, there were not quite enough of them to assure fertility. So I prescribed courses of Vitamin E & D as a placebo, this worked well. He is convinced that the administration of the drugs increased the frequency of his libido and the volume of his semen. This may be so, but he evaluates increase of semen-volume with fertility.

At the fourth examination of his semen, which contained a high sperm-count, I made him look the report for himself. That was six months ago, since when his anxiety neurosis has disappeared. He functions normally; retarded ejaculation is a thing of the past. I am convinced that if I had let him see the sperm-content of his ejaculate the first time, he would have persuaded himself that I had tricked him, and he would still be believing that he was infertile.

But it is the man or woman who enters middle age that anxiety neuroses based on sexual function become a more frequent problem. Again and again there is no physical symptom that suggests a weakening of the libido, or failure to obtain and sustain and erection in men, or the comparable responses in women. Yet the number of men and women who convince themselves that now they are growing older their sexual power has definitely begun to wane are myriad. This conviction then develops into anxiety that sooner rather than later the sex-life will end completely.

Naturally it happens that the production of sex hormones does begin to decrease, as one gets older. Only in the small fraction whose hormone production was never high, does production cease altogether. Even in old age there are sufficient quantities of the hormones present to permit full sexual activity, albeit with a lower frequency. Certainly this is so with men, and in those women where the hormone supply does peter out, the libido remains active for several years thereafter.

There is certainly no valid reason why so many men are impotent by the time they reach middle age nor why so many women become sexually unresponsive. In almost every case an anxiety neurosis centering on this fear of the loss of sexual power can be detected. The trouble is that unless professional help is sought at the onset of impotence and unresponsiveness to remove the anxiety, even a short period of both conditions can make it difficult to restore the actual physical functions. So if you find you are getting into this state of mind, seek help at once.

What I term partial impotence i.e. impotence that only occurs when the man is in a sexual situation with a woman, occurs in young men and matured men as a result of irrational anxiety. The inability to obtain or sustain an erection, or to control ejaculation, is directly caused by anxiety that the man will not be able to satisfy his partner. The counterpart of this in the women is the inability to achieve orgasm in a sexual situation with a partner, though here it is not the fear of being unable to satisfy the partner physically but the fear that by not responding physically, she will be undermining the partner's sexual confidence, so that, if he does not abandon her, he will be physically and psychologically unable to satisfy her and himself.

In the sexual situation the keynote is confidence – confidence in one's own ability to satisfy our partner's needs and our own. So long as we have this confidence, we shall never fall prey to irrational anxiety.

Chapter-17

Illnesses and Sex

Obviously, illness affects people sexually. An acute illness, which is sudden and severe, has an immediate effect. The body becomes totally involved in meeting the physical threat, and anxiety is strong until the crisis has passed and the full extent of the illness is known. Understandably, people in these circumstances have little or no energy and attention left for sexual feelings. Once the acute phase is over, most people return slowly to sexuality; but if recovery time is lengthy or if the illness results in a chronic condition, which must be lived with, there can be problems. I will discuss several of the more common condition, which may directly affect sexuality.

Heart Disease. In the forty-five-to-sixty-four-year age group the occurrence of heart disease is nearly three times as great in men as in women. After sixty-five the rates become more equalized, and it is believed the postmenopausal woman is less protected because of reduction in estrogen levels.

Heart attacks (coronary attacks) lead many people to give up sex altogether under the assumption that it will endanger their lives. Most physicians do recommend that sexual intercourse be discontinued for a period of weeks or months (roughly eight to fourteen weeks) immediately following an attack, to give healing processes plenty of time. But after that, many experts feel, sex can and should be resumed depending on the patient's interests, general fitness and conditioning. Some propose a functional test to determine when it is safe to resume: If you can walk briskly for three blocks without distress in the chest, pain, palpitations or shortness of breath, you are usually well enough for sex.

Sex can be carried out safely without sacrificing pleasure and quality. Studies tell us that, on the average, couples take ten to sixteen minutes for the sex act. The oxygen usage in sex approximates climbing one or two flights of stairs, walking rapidly at a rate of two to two and a half miles per hour, or completing many common occupational tasks. In average sexual activity the heart rate ranges from 90 to 160 beats per minute, which is the level for light to moderate physical activity. Systolic blood pressure (the upper reading, which reflects the contraction phase of the heart's action) may double from 120 to over 240, and the respiratory rate rises from 16 to 18 to about 60 breaths per minute. These 'vital signs' increase only slightly more in men than in women, perhaps due in part to the usual sexual position of the man on top. Intercourse conducted side-by-side or with the woman on top can help to reduce the exertion of the man if he is the one with the heart problem. These positions avoid sapping of energy from prolonged use of the arms and legs to support the body.

Drs. H. E. Hellerstien and E. H. Friedman studied the sexual activity of men after recovery from an acute heart attack by monitoring sexual activities in the privacy of their patients' homes. They reported that if the patient could perform exercise at levels of vigorous walking and other special activities without symptoms of abnormal pulse rate, blood pressure or ECG changes, it was generally safe to recommend the resumption of sexual activity.

It must be remembered that physical exercise leads to less likelihood of a heart attack. The sedentary person may be more prone to coronary attacks and less apt to survive the experience if one occurs. Too much food and drink before sexual intercourse can also place a strain on the heart. Of course, if the condition of the heart has deteriorated to the point that attack is imminent, it will occur with any physical exertion, not merely sex. It should also be realized that sexual arousal alone (without intercourse) affects the vital signs—although not as intensely as the sexual act itself. Finally, many everyday non-sexual activities that people are not likely to give up produce more increased heart and respiratory rates than sexual intercourse.

Impotence can follow a heart attack for both physical and psychological reasons. A man may experience chest pain (angina pectoris) during various forms of exertion, including sex that frightens him and prevents erection. To counteract this pain, coronary dilators such as nitroglycerin, prescribed by a physician, can be taken to improve circulation and reduce pain just prior to intercourse. A second common and understandable cause of impotence is fear of inducing another coronary and risking death. Yet the incidence of death during intercourse is estimated at less than one percent of sudden coronary deaths. Of this small percentage, seven out of ten deaths occur in extramarital relations, suggesting that the stressful aspects associated with such affairs, such as hurry, guilt and anxiety, are a factor.

Physicians do not always advise their patients adequately on the resumption of sexual activity after a heart attack. They may be too conservative or fail to realize the importance of sex to the patient. If you want to know more than your doctor has told you, it may be necessary to ask for specific information and directions, including a program of physical conditioning. Your sexual partner also needs to be fully informed and counseled about any changes in life style, including lovemaking, which may be necessary. *Under most circumstances there is little reason to abstain from sex after a heart attack and many reasons to continue.* Pleasure, exhilaration, release of tension, mild exercise, and a sense of well-being are some of the benefits.

Episodes of congestive heart failure are also commonly called heart attacks. When compensated by digitalis, diuretics and diet, sex is again an active possibility. Two to three weeks for recovery is advised before resuming sex. You should be able to walk briskly for three blocks without shortness of breath.

Patients with cardiac pacemakers need not give up sex. Limitations on all forms of physical activity are advised during the first two weeks following implantation to allow healing.

It is safe for most patients with heart disease due to hypertension—high blood pressure—to have sex. (Many people with hypertension have no significant impairment of heart function). Patients with average to moderate hypertension, men or women, need not restrict themselves sexually. They should, however, have their hypertension well-controlled, very severe cases of hypertension may require some modification of sexual activity; your doctor is the best judge of this.

Strokes. Strokes (cerebrovascular accidents) do not necessitate the discontinuance of sexual activity. It is extremely unlikely that further strokes can be produced through sexual exertion. If paralysis has occurred, appropriate sexual positions chosen to compensate for it can be used.

Diabetes. Sugar diabetes (diabetes mellitus) is common in late life. Most men with diabetes are not impotent, but it is one of the few illnesses, which can directly cause chronic impotence in men. Impotence occurs two to five times as often in diabetics as in the general population, even though sexual interest and desire may continue. Indeed, impotence is often the first symptom of diabetes. Most cases of diabetic-produced impotence are reversible. If the disease has been poorly controlled, there is a fair chance that proper regulation thereafter will improve potency. When impotence occurs in well-controlled diabetes, it may be permanent. (Unfortunately, if you have been diabetic for a long time, the chances are greater that the impotence will be chronic and irreversible). It is more difficult to evaluate the effects of diabetes on the sexuality of women since they do not have an obvious physical indicator like erection.

Arthritis. There are two major forms of arthritis that may cause pain during sexual activity. In rheumatoid arthritis, medications such as simple aspirin to reduce this pain and experimentation with new sexual positions, which do not aggravate pain in sensitive joints, are often helpful. A well-established program of exercise, rest and warm baths is especially useful in reducing arthritic discomfort and in facilitating sex. Indeed, much of the crippling by rheumatoid arthritis results from inactivity.

During intercourse the side-by-side position may be preferred by both men and women, especially when the patient has many tender areas and pain trigger points. Experiment until you find positions that work best for you.

There is evidence suggesting that regular sex activity helps rheumatoid arthritis, probably because of adrenal gland production of the hormone cortisone, and because of the physical activity involved. In addition, emotional stress can result from sexual dissatisfaction, and since stress worsens arthritis, sexual activity can be helpful in maintaining good functioning.

Osteoarthritis (the "wear-and-tear" disease of the joints that comes with advancing years) is usually mild and not inflammatory. This arthritis rarely interferes with sex.

Anemia. One out to four people over sixty has some measure of anemia, a common cause of fatigue and consequent reduction of sexual activity. Anemia may develop insidiously following even a mild general or localized infection, or as the result of a poor diet. Tiredness, loss of appetite and headaches are some of its early symptoms. Often an improved diet with adequate vitamins and minerals is all that is necessary to restore both energy and sexual activity.

Backache. Backache in the small of the back near the base of the spine is common among older people. Perhaps the most frequent cause is strain produced by sudden use of back muscles in a generally inactive person. In women it can be caused by osteoporosis (postmenopausal softening of the bones), related to reduction of estrogen levels. Slipped discs and arthritis are other causes of backache in both men and women.

Sufferers from arthritic backache should follow the program described above for arthritis. Sexual activity itself is an excellent form of exercise therapy for the back, stomach and pelvic muscles, and if undertaken in a regular and reasonably vigorous manner can help reduce back pain. During sex, the side position may be most comfortable if back muscles are tender. Or the backache sufferer may prefer lying on his or her back, with the partner on top. Areas of discomfort can be supported by pillows.

Hernia or Rupture. : A hernia or rupture is the protrusion of a part of the intestine through a gap or weak point in the muscular abdominal wall that contains it. The main complication to avoid is strangulation, the cutting off of the blood supply with resulting death of tissue, which is a true surgical emergency. Straining of any kind, including straining during sexual intercourse, can sometimes increase hernia symptoms such as pain and, rarely, induce strangulation. Many surgeons recommend corrective surgery early rather than waiting for an emergency to arise.

Parkinson's Disease: Parkinson's disease is a progressive nervous-system disorder of the later years marked by tremor, slowness of movement, partial facial paralysis and peculiarity of posture and gait. Depression is commonly associated with Parkinson's disease and may lead to impotence in men and lack of sexual interest in both sexes. When there is advanced organic involvement, however, impotence may be physically connected with the disease. Patients with Parkinson's disease who are treated with drugs such as L-dopa may show improved sexual performance, largely because of their generally increased sense of well being and greater mobility.

Chronic Prostatitis. Diminished sexual desire in men may be associated with chronic prostatitis. This disease is an inflammation of the prostate gland, a walnut-sized organ located just beneath the bladder in the male. It produces the milky lubricating fluid, which transports sperm during sexual intercourse. Prostatitis is characterized by a history of cloudy white discharge from the penis, usually in the morning or while straining on the toilet. Pain in the perineal region and in the end of the penis on urination and ejaculation may be present. Treatment includes antibiotics, warm sitz baths and periodic gentle prostatic massage by a physician. Sexual desire usually returns after pain lessens, especially when the pain after ejaculation eliminated.

Many doctors believe prostatitis can be caused by both too frequent and too infrequent sex. The basis for some pain between the anus and the scrotum after ejaculation may be mild prostatitis; other causes are congestion due to excessive or lengthy preliminary sexual arousal, or an unsatisfying orgasm. However, a more common cause is infrequent sex, which results in congestion in the pelvic area. Treatment in these cased consists of more frequent sexual intercourse as well as prostatic massage and warm sitz baths.

Whenever chronic prostatitis is a possibility, one should avoid excessive alcohol. Should urinary retention develop following sexual intercourse, as it occasionally does, it may be caused by the combination of a large fluid intake and the sedative effect of alcohol.

Stress Incontinence. Some women develop stress incontinence (caused by prolapse of the bladder), a condition in which there is seepage of urine because of a momentary inability to control their bladder. This happens particularly when they laugh, cough, engage in sex or otherwise exert themselves. Dyspareunia, or painful intercourse, may also be present. Stress incontinence is most frequently seen in women who have had a number of children, sometimes with unrepaired injuries following childbirth, with resulting relaxation of the supports of the uterus and bladder. It is also seen in women who have had their uterus removed surgically (hysterectomy). Slack supporting tissues may cause the bladder to protrude into the vagina (cystocele). Estrogen, taken by mouth or applied locally in the form of cream, may help firms up the vaginal lining and thus reduce the irritation from the protruding bladder. Special exercise, called Kegel's exercises are very useful. In severe cases, surgery may be required to tighten the supporting tissues.

Herniation, or prolapse of the uterus and of the rectum may occur alone or in association with prolapse. Surgical treatment is usually effective.

Excessively Enlarged Vagina. Women who have had a number of children, or difficult childbirths, or tears in the opening of the vagina at the time of childbirth may have an excessively enlarged vagina. An anterior and posterior plastic repair, a surgical procedure, may reconstruct the vagina effectively and make sex more pleasurable.

Peyronie's Disease. This disease, found in men, produces an upward bowing of the penis with the shaft angled to the right or left. A fibrous thickening of the walls of the blood vessels (corpora cavernosa) of the penis produces the symptoms, but its cause is known. Results of treatment are not predictable. Symptoms sometimes disappear spontaneously after four years or so. Intercourse can be painful and, if the penis is angled too far, impossible. However, in most cases of Peyronie's disease sex can continue. This ailment is thought to be rare, but I have seen enough of it to suspect it may be more common than is believed.

If you have had to abstain from sex for a medical reason for any length of time, some readjustment will be necessary when sexual activity is resumed. Irregular or infrequent sexual stimulation can interfere with healthy sexual functioning, adversely affecting potency in men and lubrication, vaginal shape and muscle tone in women. These difficulties are likely to taper off as activity is resumed and one should not be discouraged by initial difficulties. When a sexual partner is not available or circumstances do not permit contact with a partner, both men and women can protect much of their sexual capacity through regular masturbation, unless this is personally unacceptable.

Chapter-18

Surgery and Sex

People are understandably afraid of surgery on their sex organs. They dread possible sexual consequences in addition to the usual apprehensions aroused by any surgical procedure. Women commonly believe removal of the womb (hysterectomy) or of a breast (mastectomy) makes them "less of a woman." Men worry that prostate surgery means the end of sex life altogether. It is reassuring to know that the medical evidence does not support most of these fears.

Hysterectomy (Removal of the Womb). Technically, a hysterectomy is the removal of the womb or uterus. In addition, the ovaries and fallopian tubes may also be removed. Many hysterectomies are performed because of the presence of benign (noncancerous) tumors called fibroids, which are not troublesome so long as they remain small but may require surgery if they enlarge and produce discomfort. There is no medical evidence that careful removal of the uterus, with or without removal of the ovaries, produces any change in sexual desire or performance in women. Sexual problems are likely to be due to psychological fears: of sexual impairment, or less of femininity and attractiveness to men, or loss of sexual desire. Many women worry about premature ageing or are afraid they will develop masculine characteristics if they undergo a hysterectomy, but there is no basis for these worries.

There can be pain during sex (dyspareunia) if intercourse is resumed up to four weeks after hysterectomy, due to incomplete healing in the vagina. Except for this temporary discomfort, a hysterectomy has no effect on any part of the vagina involved in intercourse. Though the cervix is no longer present at the far end of the vagina, this does not affect the sexual act or desire. In women who have not yet completed the menopause and have children as they want, sexual desire can actually increase after surgery because pregnancy is no longer a concern. If the ovaries are removed, loss of estrogen may bring changes in the lining of the vagina, but, as we have noted, this is treatable. Removal of the ovaries after menopause generally produces far fewer direct symptoms than removal before menopause because the ovaries have already stopped functioning or show a substantial reduction in estrogen output. On the other hand, removal of all or parts of a woman's childbearing apparatus, powerful symbols of womanhood, often does have significant psychological effects. If the woman sees this surgery as symbolic "castration," she needs to resolve this, either on her own or with outside help. She must understand that removal does not eradicate sexuality, cause unattractiveness or diminish her womanliness.

Mastectomy (Breast Removal). While most breast lumps are found to be benign, unfortunately the likelihood of breast cancer increases with age. Breast removal, or mastectomy, is performed when a lump in the breast is found to be malignant (cancerous). There are different kinds of mastectomies, ranging from removal of the lump and some adjacent tissue only to the removal of the entire breast, surrounding lymph glands and chest muscles. Although these operations can be lifesaving, they have understandable psychological implications for many women because they not only change the outward appearance of the body but also visibly alter a specific symbol of sexuality. Breast removal can actually be more difficult to adjust to than a hysterectomy, which leaves no obvious signs beyond an abdominal scar. Although there is no physiological change in sexual capacity after mastectomy, women may temporarily lose their sexual desire out of embarrassment, their inability to accept the loss of the breast, and fear that they have become less attractive to their sexual partners. They are afraid the absence of the breast will be noticeable in public. A properly fitting prosthetic bra can relieve worries about public appearance, but reactions to breast loss by women themselves and their partners are not always so easily resolved.

Men, too, need a period of adjustment to work out their feelings about breast surgery in their partners. In sturdy relationships, time and affection often take care of disturbed feelings following breast removal. Severe and prolonged negative reactions may require professional psychotherapy.

Prostatectomy (Removal of the prostate Gland). As men get older, up to half of them will experience inflammation or enlargement of the prostate. At least half of these will require surgery. When the enlargement is noncancerous, as is usually the case, it is called benign prostatic hypertrophy (B.P.H).

The causes of prostatic difficulties are unknown but may be connected to changes in hormone levels. There is no foundation to the common folklore that prostate trouble is related to "excessive" sexual activity. Indeed, evidence suggests that an active sex life preserves healthy prostate functioning.

Since the prostate gland is so close to the bladder, its enlargement causes it to push up against the bladder or urethra, usually producing problems with urination. An enlarged prostate may increase the need to urinate or to get up to void during the night. There may be a delay in starting the stream of urine, or even a total inability to urinate. Enlargement of the gland tends to occur slowly, and because it leads to retention and stagnation of urine there can be bacterial infection. In severe and untreated cases, damage is done to the kidneys. Surgery is absolutely necessary when a urinary shutdown occurs. Some doctors now recommend surgery at an earlier point in the course of symptoms to avoid unnecessary complications and dire emergencies.

Three types of surgery, all requiring anaesthesia, are used:

Transurethral resection, or TUR. This is the commonest and least traumatic procedure because it requires no outside incision. A thin Bakelite or plastic sheath is inserted in the penis, a tungsten wire is maneuvered through the tube, and the gland is removed. The tissue sometimes grows back following TUR. TUR is recommended chiefly when the prostate is not too enlarged, or for men after seventy.

Suprapubic. If the gland is very large, an incision is made through the abdomen to remove the tissue.

Perineal. This procedure is recommended for men with substantial prostate enlargement who, because of advanced age or physical condition, are unable to withstand the stress of prolonged anaesthesia. It can be performed with relative safety even on a very elderly man. An incision is made between the scrotum and anus (the perineum), removing most or the entire prostate.

Potency is rarely affected by the TUR and suprapubic procedures, and some men actually experience increased potency because their prostatic symptoms have been eliminated. The perineal approach—especially the radical procedure—is the chief physical cause of impotence following prostatic surgery. (Some doctors feel only the radical procedure may have this effect.)

Prior to surgery prostate problems usually do not interfere with sexual functioning unless pain is present. After a prostatectomy, as we have noted, most men return to normal sexual activity. Healing time runs at last six weeks. The only change after surgery is that semen is no longer ejaculated through the opening of the penis but instead pushes backward into the bladder (retrograde ejaculation), where it is voided with the urine. This so-called dry ejaculation happens because a space has been left where the enlarged prostate had been, and fluid travels the path of least resistance to the bladder. Although men are then no longer able to father children, the large majority have erections as before, with no diminishment of sexual pleasure. In some cases even the ejaculation from the penis returns following some regrowth of the prostate; in such instances, fertility may be restored.

By far the greatest cause of impotence occurring with prostatectomies is psychological. This impotence is frequently reversible. The fear is based on the tendency to associate the prostate gland with the penis since men know the two are located physically close to each other. Unfortunately, family doctors and urologists do not always give a man adequate information about what to expect after surgery, so that he falsely assumes sexual impairment.

Orchidectomy (Removal of the Testes). This surgery may be performed because of cancer of the testes. The psychological impact of such castration can be devastating. Emotional preparation before surgery and counseling following surgery are indispensable.

Colostomy and Ileostomy (Removal of Sections of the Intestine). When part of the bowel (large intestine) must be removed for lifesaving purposes, the anus is closed and an artificial opening in the abdomen is created. The surgery may be in the colon (colostomy) or in the ileum (an ileostomy). Needless to say, the patient has many sensitive adjustments to make after such surgery. A bag is attached to the opening. This bag fills with feaces and must be emptied. There are embarrassing bowel sounds as well as odors. Much of this can be controlled adequately. Patients will have to work their way through their own feelings, however, as well as their perception of other people's attitudes. The most complicated issue of all can be the working out of the sexual relationship with one's partner. Patients who had active sex lives prior to ostomies usually continue to do so afterward, but inevitably there is a complex adjustment process, and you and your partner should not hesitate to seek help.

In general, for both men and women, the emotionally charged aspects of surgery which affects sex can be relatively short-lived if people spell out their fears and if their misconceptions are cleared up. Unfortunately, they often do not get the opportunity to do this. Doctors do not always take the time to explain procedures and answer questions, though counseling before surgery is extremely helpful in preventing anxiety and clarifying misunderstandings. After the operation, continued advice and emotional support from medical personnel, family and friends and special organizations are crucial to adjustment.

Even under the best of modern techniques, rates of recovery vary with the individual after surgery of any kind. Some people will find their stamina or vitality reduced for some time, even though healing has been satisfactory. Surgeons do not always make it clear to their patients that these are normal variations. You have no reason to worry if this happens to you, as long as your surgeon has assured you that your postoperative recovery is progressing, as it should. Once you are feeling entirely well again, your level of sexual activity will return to normal.

Chapter-19

Menstruation

Menstruation is periodic bleeding from the womb via the vagina in women of childbearing age. It is also known by a variety of other terms e.g. the Period, the Monthlies, and the Curse.

Menstruation denotes the onset of puberty in the girl, and the first menstruation (known as the menarche)may appear between the ages of 9 and 12, though 12 is the average age. Most girls have had their menarche by the age of 15, but if a girl has not menstruated by 13, a doctor should be consulted. He will be able to diagnose whether the non-appearance of the menarche is due to physical underdevelopment, which will right itself in time, or to a hormone disturbance, which can be treated at once by the administration of a hormone or hormones. Treatment of the failure to begin menstruating should never be attempted except under medical supervision.

Menstruation continues at regular intervals until the woman reaches the menopause (change of life) usually between 50 and 55. After the menopause, which is a gradual process that may take up to three or fours years to complete, the woman never again menstruates, and is no longer capable of becoming pregnant.

The average length of the menstrual cycle is 28 days. There are some women, however, who have cycles of 26, 27, 29, 30 and 31 days.

Menstruation is the result of several processes taking place in the woman's reproductive system. Every woman is born with roughly 800,000 immature eggs divided between her two ovaries. In each menstrual cycle an egg develops. It reaches maturity mid-way in the menstrual cycle and is released into the Fallopian tube. (The ovaries take it in turn to release the eggs). It is now capable of being fertilized by a male sperm. If the egg is not fertilized in about 48 hours it begins to degenerate, and moves down the Fallopian tube towards the womb.

Meanwhile, the lining of the womb has been building up a highly enriched blood supply, with which to receive the fertilized egg. The fertilized egg will embed itself in the lining of the womb and begin to develop into an embryo and the menstruation would not occur. If it has not been fertilized, however, the lining of the womb becomes detached and passed out of the womb through the vagina, along with the collected blood and which is then called menstruation. The process in the next month then begins all over again.

The length of the blood-flow varies from individual to individual. The average is between 3 and 5 days. Bleeding that continues for more than 6 days should receive medical attention.

For most women, menstruation causes no trouble, beyond the rather messy business of disposing of blood-soaked sanitary napkins or tampons. There are other women, however, who are regularly plagued with headaches, backache and stomachache, tender swollen breasts and other symptoms in the two or three days before menstruation begins. Others experience pain throughout the period of the flow.

The menstrual cycle can be interrupted or otherwise affected by a variety of causes. Illness, even the common cold, can upset it completely, or for a few days. So can all kinds of emotional tensions, depression and anxiety.

Delay in the beginning of a period by no means indicates that the woman is pregnant.

Any woman who experiences excessive bleeding or bleeding between periods should immediately consult a doctor. Modern medical science has now the means of treating most, if not all, menstrual disorders, and no woman should fail to make use of them.

I am often asked whether making love during menstruation can cause any physical harm to the woman. There is no medical reason whatsoever why lovemaking should not be continued throughout menstruation; it has no harmful effects either on the woman or the man. The only possible objections could come from the man on aesthetic grounds; and, naturally, cunnilingus will have to be omitted from foreplay should the man object.

It is widely thought among laymen that conception cannot result from intercourse during menstruation. Though it is not a common occurrence, it can happen, so to be on the safe side a contraceptive should be used, unless the woman has been fitted with and IUD. The most convenient contraceptive is the French letter, since diaphragms and cervical caps must not be used during menstruation.

For some women, the flow is a steady one from its first appearance and is so every time. Other women are occasional 'slow-starters' i.e. the flow begins with small trickles of blood released at intervals during the first couple of days; while as many more are habitual 'slow-starters' experience an unpleasant kind of physical congestion, or an emotional uneasiness.

It has been discovered that if a 'slow-starters' makes love, and her partner is careful to arouse her so that she has a really intense orgasm, the contractions of the womb during orgasm speed up the flow, and relieve her of her physical and psychological tensions.

A nuisance though menstruation undoubtedly is from a social point of view, and has been well-named. The Curse, it must be treated as a normal biological process. A woman who considers herself to be sick, and takes to her bed or cuts down on her usual activities during menstruation, is making the experience much worse than it need to be.

Chapter-20

The Menopause

The menopause literally means 'the cessation of the menses' (monthly periods). Sometimes it is referred to as the 'climacteric' or 'the Change of Life'.

It does not take place overnight, but over a period that can vary in different women from less than a year to four or five years. When it is complete, the ovaries no longer produce mature eggs, the lining of the womb remains unchanged, and the menstrual cycle, culminating in menstruation itself, comes to an end. The woman is no longer capable of bearing children.

During the menopause, the changes mentioned above take place gradually. At the beginning menstruation becomes irregular, and continues to be more and more irregular until it ceases altogether.

The menopause usually begins between the ages of 45 and 50. There are cases in which women in their late thirties experience it, and others in which the process has not begun until the middle fifties. There are statistics which show that women who began to menstruate early, between 10 and 12, are late in beginning the menopause, while those who did not begin to menstruate until 15, 16 or 17 are over the menopause by the time they reach their fourties.

The early stopping of the menstrual flow need not necessarily indicate the beginning of the menopause. It can be the result of disease, especially anaemia, or of a hormonal dysfunction, known as amenorrhea, which causes consecutive periods to be missed. The woman who misses her periods early should always have a medical check-up to determine whether the cause is disease or hormonal dysfunction, or the true onset of the menopause.

One of the chief factors in producing the changes in ovaries and womb is the slowing down of he production of the female sex-hormone oestrogen, which has a number of functions. It is partly responsible for the woman's sexual desire, it tones up the lining of the vagina, preventing soreness during intercourse, and it promotes mineralization of bone, loss of which results in aches in the bones and joints, irritation of the bladder and incontinence of urine.

The ovaries also produce other female sex hormones; follicle stimulating hormone (FHS), which causes the egg to develop in the follicle, and the follicle to burst and release the egg; and progesterone, which prepares the lining of the womb to receive the fertilized egg. The ovaries cease production of FHS and progesterone fairly early in the menopause, but stop the production of oestrogen more gradually. In fact, after the menopause has been completed, the ovaries often continue to produce a small amount of oestrogen for some years.

During the years before the menopause, the ovaries are stimulated to produce their hormones by the hypophysis or pituitary gland. The hypophysis, which is the size of a small nut, and is situated just beneath the brain, is often referred to as the master gland, because it regulates the functions of all the other endocrine glands. As one grows older, the hypophysis produces smaller and smaller quantities of the hormones that stimulate the ovaries into producing their hormones. However, when the ovaries are no longer producing oestrogen, the hypophysis encourages the production of sex-stimulating hormones by the outer portions of the adrenal glands. Thus, in most women, the libido continues to function after the ovaries have ceased to produce oestrogen. But if the libido does disappear during the menopause, it can now be restored by very small controlled does of the male sex hormone, testosterone.

Symptoms

In the past, women regarded the menopause with mixed feelings. On the one hand, when it was over, the monthly period of discomfort would be a thing of the past, and the fear of pregnancy would be gone for ever; while on the other, there were the four or five years of suffering and possible danger to life itself, which, it was believed, were the inevitable accompaniment of the 'Change'.

Nowadays, the suffering and possible danger to life is themselves, happily, things of the past.

Four-fifths of all women go through the menopause without suffering any ill effects, and, as far as their general health is concerned, they are scarcely aware of the changes that are taking place, beyond the increasing irregularity of menstruation; for the remaining one-fifth, even they have the symptoms in a mild from if the psychological approach is good; and because modern medicine is able to treat the symptoms, they do not have to put up with any discomfort, if they will consult their doctor.

In other words, every woman should be able to take the menopause in her stride, as the natural process that it is. In the majority of case where the symptoms are very pronounced, the discomfort they create can be alleviated by medication, sometimes aided by psychotherapy.

Without doubt, the best known of all the menopausal symptoms are the *hot flushes*. What causes hot flushes is this. In the walls of the small arteries near the surface of the skin, there are muscles and nerves. Some of the nerves constrict the arteries so that the blood in them is forced elsewhere and the skin becomes pale; other dilate the vessels so that blood can flow into them. The hormone changes which take place during the menopause affect the tone to these blood vessels, so that the dilator nerves often over-power, as it were, the constrictor nerves. The result is flushing of the face, head and neck, and a sensation of heat throughout the body.

Hot flushes happen suddenly, without warning. Sometimes they are so severe that they make the sufferer sweat, and this can cause embarrassment. But no matter how severe the attacks are, the doctor can quickly and successfully treat them.

A general sense of tiredness sometimes so acute that the sufferer feels exhausted, probably takes the menopausal woman more often to the doctor's consulting-room than any other symptom. The woman does not feel like this every day, because the ovaries do not suddenly stop functioning. In this case, the slowing down results in temporary changes in the blood vessels and nerves, which normally give the body its energy.

This symptom, too, can be successfully treated, but it must be pointed out that not all the tiredness felt by the menopausal woman is necessarily caused by the menopausal changes. Tiredness and feelings of exhaustion are the symptoms of many diseases. The doctor must examine the patient thoroughly to determine that any of the diseases –among which are vitamin deficiency, anaemia, diabetes, tuberculosis, and adrenal gland failure – are not present before he treats for menopausal fatigue.

Women going through the 'change' often complain of sleeplessness. They may find it difficult to fall asleep, or they may wake up in the early hours and be unable to sleep again. This menopausal insomnia is caused by the hormonal and other changes taking place in the body, and it is unwise for the sufferer to try to improve her condition by taking sleeping pills. Instead she should consult her doctor, who will prescribe the right treatment.

'Aches and pains all over', though sometimes located in a specific area of the body e.g. the neck, the base of the skull, in the joints and in the chest, is another common symptom. As with fatigue, 'aches and pains' are the symptoms of other diseases besides the menopause, and a medical examination must be carried out to make sure that they actually are the result of the menopause. The administration of small doses of hormones to make up for the hormone deficiency created by the changing ovaries can eliminate this symptom.

Some women complain of having more frequent headaches during the 'Change', others of palpitations, difficulty in breathing, lack of concentration, loss of appetite, increased frequency of urination, strange tingling sensations in the skin and suchlike experiences. If these symptoms are more real than imaginary, they are unlikely to be the result of menopausal changes. The doctor should be consulted, nevertheless.

Perhaps the most frightening of the menopausal symptoms is what is known as 'flooding '. Without warning, there may be a fairly heavy vaginal discharge of blood, which takes the victim unawares. It is caused by the irregularities in the menstrual cycle, which the changes within the body are bringing about. If it happens once, the woman goes in constant fear that it may happen again. If she visits her doctor after her first experience, he will see that she never has another.

Finally there are a number of women who are very much disturbed by feelings of irritability and anxiety. They are usually women who have been of a nervous disposition for a number of years. As they approach the age when the menopause is likely to overtake them, this nervousness increases, and the realization that the 'Change' has at last begun increases their anxiety and leads to irritability. Few of the other symptoms affect anyone but the sufferer herself, but irritability, if it is not checked by treatment, can cause unhappiness and distress to the other members of the family. The latter can do much to help by their understanding and extra kindness during this time.

Let me repeat: Four-fifths of all women would be unaware that they were going through the menopause were it not for the irregularity of their menstrual periods. Those who do have any of the symptoms described above, should not hesitate to go to their doctors, who can invariably treat them successfully.

Sex and the Menopause

The four-fifths of women who take the menopause in their stride, and have few if any ill effects from it, are almost invariably women who have previously had fully satisfactory and satisfying sex-lives, and see no reason why they should not continue to make love as usual despite the changes that are taking place in their bodies. If the women do have difficulties could persuade themselves, or be persuaded, that a full and active sex-life is as important a part of any treatment that the doctor prescribes, there would be far fewer than one-fifth who would suffer discomfort to any degree at this time.

There are two main psychological approaches to the menopause and sex. There are the woman who have gone through their lives up to this point with a fear, shame or disgust of sex, who have hated every sexual contact they have ever had, These women seize on the menopause as an excuse for stopping all sexual activity, and are doomed to an unrewarding old age.

The woman's ability to achieve orgasm *is in no way affected by the menopause,* and happily there are many who, realizing this, realize also that the menopause will remove forever the possibility of their ever becoming pregnant again. Quite a number of women who have made use of a reliable contraceptive, including some who have been on the Pill, have never been able to rid themselves entirely of the fear of unwanted pregnancy, and this fear, even when not a very conscious one, has prevented them from enjoying their lovemaking one hundred per cent.

With the fear of pregnancy definitely and permanently removed by the completion of the menopause, these women determine to enjoy sex as they have never enjoyed it before. As I pointed out earlier, the production of oestrogen by the ovaries plays an important part in regulating the woman's sexual desire. Fortunately the production of oestrogen by the ovaries tails off very very gradually, and quite a number of years pass after the completion of the menopause before it ceases altogether. Logically, as the oestrogen production slows down, so the frequency of the woman's sexual desire ought to decrease. However, those women who make up their minds to take on a new lease of sex-life after the menopause often find their new experience far different from their earlier experience of making of love.

Many a husband has been surprised, and some even alarmed, by the frequency of the demands for sex their post-menopausal wives make. Not only does her sexual desire function more frequently, but also she loses many of her former inhibitions. Some husbands have claimed that their post-menopausal wives have become sexually totally unrecognizable.

Any man who finds himself in this happy situation should have no hesitation in making the most of it. Unhappily, by the time this happens, many men have let their own sex-lives deteriorate. Since the husband is generally a year or two older than the wife, he may be approaching sixty when these new demands are made on him, and for the last ten years he has been devoting most of his tailing-off energies to his work and has let sex take an inferior place in his life. He may find it difficult to obtain a full erection, which makes penetration far from easy, if possible at all; he may have developed premature ejaculation because he has lost the knack of controlling his speed to orgasm.

Confronted with the middle-aged wife and her newfound zest for sex, he may panic and become totally impotent, because he fears that he may never be able to satisfy her. But instead of panicking, he should sit down with her, quietly reassess their situation. With patience, persistence and the willing co-operation of the wife, coupled with the sincere desire of the husband to function normally again, an entirely new and exciting sexual experience can be moulded. Together they may spend the closing phases of their lives in an intimacy that, no matter how satisfying their early sexual experience was, adds a quality to living they had not thought of before.

Chapter-21

Alcohol and Sex

Alcohol is the term applied to a large group of colorless Liquid compound all of which are poisonous to some extent. When the layman refers to alcohol, however, he is referring to one of the compounds only and though he may not know that its name is ethyl alcohol, he drinks it (with pleasure) in the guise of whiskey, gin, vodka, brandy, liqueurs, wines, aperitives, and beer.

Ethyl alcohol is produced by the fermenting action of yeast on cereals, potatoes and fruits. The 'potency' of an alcoholic drink is gauged in terms of alcoholic content, to which the term 'proof' is given. A 100% proof spirit, for example, contains about 50 per cent alcohol.

Alcoholic drinks are divided into four categories: spirits and liqueurs (whiskey, gin, vodka, brandy and the whole range of liqueurs) which are usually between 50° and 70° proof (all good brands of whiskey, gin and vodka are 70° proof); fortified wines and aperitives, such as sherry and port, and the wide range of aperitives, which are fortified with pure alcohol or brandy, and contain between 16 and 18 per cent alcohol; wines, which usually have a 7 to 15 percent alcohol content; and beers, which have a 5 per cent alcohol content.

Alcohol is a food, something like sugar. It is cram-full with calories, but it does not provide any of the nutrients the body needs. As soon as it comes into contact with the lining of the stomach, it is absorbed into the bloodstream. For this reason, alcohol drunk during or after a meal is absorbed more slowly than alcohol drunk on an 'empty stomach'.

As soon as it enters the bloodstream, it is carried to the liver, then to the heart, the lungs and the brain. Having reached the brain it slows down it's activity and impairs the efficiency of the central nervous system. Worries and inhibitions are discarded, and the drinker goes through a phase of carefree exhilaration and happiness.

This phase marks what might be termed the beneficial effects of alcohol.

However, be all that as it may, it is a fact that in the concentration of one per cent, alcohol acts like an anaesthetic on the brain and the nervous system. Perception and the thought processes are further slowed down. It becomes difficult to co-ordinate movement, and the ability to react quickly is lost. If you persist in drinking after you have become drunk, and the concentration of alcohol builds up, after a certain point the alcohol has a poisoning effect. The body reacts with nausea and vomiting, and in extreme cases unconsciousness, from which the drinker emerges with a rageing headache, an upset stomach, and other symptoms of hangover.

Alcohol taken in moderate quantities is a good pick-me-up. It is when it is habitually taken to excess that it becomes really dangerous, for it results in a condition known as chronic alcoholism, in which drinking becomes compulsive with the same effect as addiction to drugs. The alcoholic is unable to control his desire for drink, and will go to amazing and cunning lengths to see that he has a supply of alcohol always at hand.

Chronic alcoholism, to which both sexes are susceptible, is nowadays regarded as an illness, which, indeed, it is. There is evidence to suggest that some cases are the result of a defect in the body's metabolism, i.e. the process whereby food and drink is converted into new living matter and waste. This metabolic defect results in the body using alcohol in a way that makes it more poisonous than it is to people who do not have the defect.

Whether this metabolic malfunction is congenital or whether it is induced by constant excessive drinking is not at present known, but there are a very large number of cases of chronic alcoholism which are the result of a clearly traceable progression from 'social drinking' to 'problem drinking' to addiction.

The trouble with alcohol is that the more one drinks, the more one builds up a tolerance to its effects, with the result that eventually one needs to take more and more to produce the desired effects. The frequent social drinker is, therefore, always in danger, even if he controls his intake of alcohol during one session, of developing this tolerance and the progressive need for more alcohol, which eventual becomes compulsion.

When this stage is reached personality changes occur. The former frank and trusting man or woman becomes suspicious and resentful, and these traits are increased if the alcoholic is criticized or rejected by family and friends. The appetite declines, resulting in an unbalanced diet, which undermines the general health. In the last stages, the liver, heart, and nerves are affected, which may lead to convulsions and delirium tremens and eventual death.

The same fate awaits the man or woman who takes to the bottle to forget problems and anxieties, which seem too much for them to cope with. This reason for drinking postulates character already present when the drinker began to comfort himself by blocking out the anxiety or problem from the consciousness with alcohol. This type of cause of chronic alcoholism probably occurs more often than the chronic alcoholism derived from over-frequent social drinking. But whatever the cause, the end results are the same.

There is only one cure for chronic alcoholism – absolute abstention from taking alcohol in any form for the rest of one's life. This, of course, is a drastic remedy, and one, which the compulsion and addiction of the disease makes a cure possible only if the alcoholic can somehow be encouraged in his desire to be cured.

There are a number of treatments available, but they have to be specially tailored to the individual needs of the patient. For example, when anxiety and depression have caused the compulsion, a sedative may relieve these states of mind, and so remove the compulsion. For other cases, there are various drugs, which work on the principle of aversion therapy. Taken with alcohol, they make the latter taste so horrible and have other extremely unpleasant effects, that the patient develops a thorough loathing for it.

But as I have said, no matter what the initial cause of the disease, every chronic alcoholic has an underlying psychiatric disorder. The first step should, therefore, always be to consult a psychiatrist or doctor who specializes in treating the illness, so that an exact diagnosis may be obtained of the precise needs of the patient.

As may be imagined from what I have said so far, since the brain and general nervous system are rapidly affected by alcohol, it is inevitable that the highly sensitive sexual nervous system, which relies so heavily on the brain for its proper functioning, is also affected. It goes without saying that the majority of chronic alcoholics are impotent men or frigid women.

Both sexes have suffered a striking decline in the frequency of their sexual desire, and in their sexual capacity and performance. In my view, then, it is safe to say, that to embark on a course of heavy drinking is an almost cast-iron guarantee for making oneself sexually defective. It is a pity that alcohol should be abused in this way, because taken in the right doses; it can enhance the sexual experience, chiefly by removing anxiety and inhibitions, and help to overcome certain male dysfunctions, especially too rapid ejaculation which it does by desensitizing the orgasm-producing nerves, and female dysfunction, mainly delayed orgasm, which it operates by freeing the woman of her inbred feelings of guilt, sin or shame.

Chapte-22

How You Began Life

Some amazing fact and figures about the miracle of conception

The tiny, threadlike cell, which the male produces to create a new life, was first recognized under the microscope almost three hundred years ago—in 1677. Though much information about the sperm has since been amassed by scientific workers in the field, some questions still cannot be answered by most ordinarily well informed persons. How many individuals, for example, still believe in the ancient fiction that young men must take care not to waste their sexual secretions, but to "save themselves" for the future?

Actually we know that sperms are supplied in an almost never-ending quantity to the normal male, and like saliva, are not "used up." This despite the fact that a single emission of normal semen (the sperm plus secretions furnished by various glands) contains from 400 to 500 million sperm, or spermatozoa! Obviously, to accomplish this task, the glands which produce these sperm—the testicles (egg-shaped glands situated in the scrotum)—must have a highly complicated structure. The testicles produce the sperm in about 300 sections of microscopic tubes, known as *seminiferous tubules.* Uncoiled, the network of tubes in the testicles extends almost a mile. Surprisingly, the normal temperature of the human body is too high for sperm production. For this reason, Nature has provided the scrotum outside the body, a bag with its own mechanism to regulate temperature. One of the methods, which regulate temperature, is the action of a special muscle. When the temperature is low, this muscle contracts to bring the testicles closer to the warmth of the body. When it is hot, the muscle lowers the scrotum away from the body. The result is a scrotal temperature that is five to ten degrees (Centigrade) lower than body temperature. These facts have let doctors to advise men who have a fertility problem to take special precautions. While most men retain full fertility even though they take prolonged hot baths or Turkish baths, some men of low fertility might suffer impaired sperm production from these practices and are advised to avoid them. It is also advisable for men with a fertility problem not to wear tight-fitting underwear or trousers.

The average person is under the impression that, when ejaculation occurs, sperm are ejected directly from the testicles. This is not since the sperm have a long trip to make before they reach the point of ejaculation. They must first travel from the tubes where they are produced, to the tail of the coiled tube known as the *epididymis*—a 20-foot trip that may require two weeks. From there they must traverse the eighteen-inch length of the sperm duct-a trip whose time has not yet been entirely established. However, we do know that sperm have been found in the ejaculate as long as five or six weeks after the sperm ducts have been cut—which means that these sperm could not have come from the testicles but must have been lodged somewhere along the sperm ducts above the point cut. How vast is the journey the sperm must take can be judged when one realizes the size of the average sperm—it must traverse 500 times its own length just to travel one inch. Each inch can be compared to a man's swimming one mile. Propelled by its hair-like tail, this tiny germ cell carries a cargo of at least 30,000 genes, each of which determines the kind of inheritance a child will have if the sperm is successful in reaching its distant goal—the female egg. Some years ago it was believed that before ejaculation, the sperm and semen were stored in the seminal vesicles. Most research opinion today holds that sperms are not normally found in these vesicles. However, a recent experiment was conducted where semen was collected in four separate fractions, the last being the secretion from the vesicles. Since the experimenter found in this last secretion a number of degenerated sperm, he concluded that sperm were present in variable but often large numbers in the vesicles. Other experimenters found some years ago that 75 per cent of the sperm are found in the first 40 per cent of the normal ejaculate. They concluded that, just before ejaculation, sperms are concentrated at a point close to the ejaculatory duct in what is known as the *ampulla.*

The normal environment of the sperm is alkaline—acid is deadly to it. Yet surprisingly the female vagina is strongly acid. This may be Nature's way of stirring the sperm into greater effort to reach the more alkaline conditions of the womb. Most sperm do not live more than a few hours after ejaculation, generally up to twelve, rarely more than thirty, though some have been known to last as long as 72 hours in their search for the egg. The usual site of fertilization is the midpoint in the fallopian tube. On rare occasions the sperm will meet the egg at some other point in the body, with the result being a type of ectopic (out of place) pregnancy which must be ended by the physician. The exact method by which sperm reach the fallopian tubes is still not established. The sperm do possess the ability to move, but experimental work with animals indicates that this may not be the chief means of transport. Work done with cows revealed that muscular contractions of the womb during copulation might aid in this process. It has also been shown that the hormone oxytocin stimulates womb contractions and accelerates the transportation of the sperm in these animals. Work with humans has, for obvious reasons, been very scanty, but the same factors may operate. It has been suggested that contractions at the time of orgasm may help to pull semen through the womb mouth into the womb. There is also evidence that oxytocin may be released by the female at the time of orgasm.

The estimate has been made that human spermatozoa, by their own efforts, can move at a rate of 3 mm (about 1/10th of an inch) per minute through the female reproductive tract. At this rate, it should taken a sperm a minimum of three-quarters of an hour in the average woman to travel from the womb mouth to the point in the tube where fertilization occurs. However, recent experiments on women have shown that other factors may make it possible for much more rapid transportation of sperm to take place. These experiments were preformed on three women about to undergo abdominal hysterectomy at about the time of ovulation. Just before the surgery, carbon particles were placed in the vagina of the women (who were under anaesthesia) and at the same time, oxytocin was injected. **In two of the women, carbon particles were found in the tubes**

28 and 34 minutes later. These data supported the belief that contractions of the womb, aided by oxytocin may play an important part in transportation, since the carbon particles obviously had no mobility of their own. One of the most recent findings, reported only during the last year, has been the dramatic discovery that there is an obvious difference between the head of the sperm which carries a Y chromosome (resulting in a male when fertilization takes place) and the sperm, which carries an X chromosome (resulting in a female when fertilization takes place). The first had a smaller, round-headed shape; the second had a larger, oval-headed shape.

Even when a sperm does fertilize an egg, there is no guarantee that the fertilized egg will develop to maturity and produce a live-offspring. It has been concluded that the proportion of fertilized eggs that perish before birth is about 30 per cent for animals and probably as high for humans. It is well known that abnormally shaped sperm are associated with infertility. It is not established to what extent these abnormal sperm are capable of fertilizing an egg if they do have an opportunity. The best opinion holds that chances of these sperms being able to penetrate an egg—even if they managed to reach the site of fertilization—would be very low. When one realizes how very complicated is this "story of the sperm," one is not surprised to learn that perhaps 10 million couples are childless against their will, with the reason found in some deficiency in the male sperm or male reproductive tract in almost half the cases. **It is to be hoped that—out of the expanding volume of research in this field—will soon come a happier ending to the story for those couples now denied a child.**

Chapter-23

Sex Stimulants

The advertising pages of magazines of a certain type are filled with offerings of various patent medicines, foods and appliances "guaranteed to stimulate faltering potency. In any field of commercial life the total sales can be estimated by the amount spent in advertising. In this case, then, millions of Rupees must be spent yearly by men for medicines to increase their sexual prowess. As far as real value is concerned or actual benefit derived, every Rupee spent in this direction is a Rupee wasted. An *aphrodisiac* is some agent used to stimulate the sexual response. It need not be a drug or a food—it may be simply an impression received by any of the senses. Whatever it is, the effect produced is more often mental than physical. **This is really main idea back of all the patent medicines. If a man pays out real money for even bread pills, and has faith in them, that faith may act as a tonic, if he is still able to respond to a tonic.** So, in a broad sense, any impression creating a desire for sexual intercourse is an aphrodisiac. At present the human race is living in a world surrounded by such impressions. The movies we see, the magazines sold at news-stands, the dresses of the woman with whom one comes in contact, in fact, much of our everyday life stimulates sexual desire. The normal human being who has wisely used his body needs no aphrodisiacs other than those that come his way as easily as the sunshine and the warm breezes of summer. Hunger for food creates a desire; hunger for air causes a repetition of respiratory breathing; cold makes clothing necessary, while heat brings a desire for lighter covering. **A normal man does not have to spend money for drugs to tell him when to eat or to put on an overcoat. Similarly, a normal man can go through all the decades of adult existence and be perfectly happy without spending a moment's thought or a Rupee of money on the matter of so-called aphrodisiacs.** But, with the tried, anxious individual whose potency is diminishing, the problem is different. Nothing frightens him more than the so-called "loss of manhood." He feels that it is the first and the greatest step towards an early grave. The greater the worry, the more pronounced is the weakness. The more the despair, the harder is the struggle to recall the physical ability of youth. While the greatest benefit would be derived from complete rest, such men struggle all the harder to prove themselves. Grasping at every straw, they spend their money for every new nostrum they see advertised. *Unfortunately, nothing helps: they fail to include the greatest of all medicines—complete rest.*

In the early days of electricity, a Frenchman brought over to England an electrical bed. It was an elegant couch, with many bright wires running above it. The bed, the room and the mattress were supposed to be charged with electricity that would enter the body of the man sleeping on it and give him strength and power. No matter to what degree a man was impotent, he was told he could use that bed one night and he would produce a son. The price per night was 500 Pounds. The bed was to remain in England only a certain number of nights. Needless to say, it was well occupied. Every man was either satisfied or was ashamed to say that he was not; and the French fraud returned to his home, months before any of the victims could tell whether they were to become parents or not. This is an example of the fraud behind all aphrodisiacs. Today they exist by the dozen, and they all have behind them the false hope that, if something is done to the human body, something will happen. They are all physiologically wrong, and, at the best, are simply goads to the jaded horse who is trying to pull the burden to the top of the hill and be alive when he reaches it. The proper treatment for that tired horse is to take his harness off and let him rest, instead of stimulating him with whip and spur. Medical aphrodisiacs can be divided into two classes: first, those that are composed of harmless substances, which, while they do no harm, are equally unable to do any good. *A man taking such pills by the hundred suffers no harm except to his pocketbook.* Failure of one brand to act simply leads him to another. *The other group comprises combinations of drugs that, taken in excess, are powerful poisons.* Foremost among the agents that have been used for this purpose is *strychnine*—a stimulant in small amounts, though a well-known deadly poison in quantities. Another drug, similar in nature and source, is *brucine. Atropine* is also used as well as *ergotin. Cocaine* was used, until it fell into disrepute for its habit-forming qualities. In Italy, *quinine* was once favored. *Cantharides* ("Spanish fly") is spoken of by the uneducated, and half-educated, as a sure inspirer of sexual power; it is a corrosive poison, which blisters even the skin. *Phosphorous,* also a powerful poison, was often prescribed; phosphates and hypophosphites are still in general use for many types of fatigued conditions. Drugs may indeed whip the jaded appetite, but their end results are more deadly than the condition that they are supposed to cure. Those acting directly on the *genito-urinary* system are irritants, excreted through the urine. Given in large amounts, they inflame the tract from the kidneys down to the urethra. This irritation may end in haemorrhage, suppression of urine, and even death. **The situation resolves itself into a simple summary. Aphrodisiacs that are harmless are worthless; those that are potent are desperately dangerous. Let the buyer beware! He buys at his own risk.**

Chapter-24

A New Cure for the Impotent Male

Penile implants—placing silicone rods inside the penis—are helping many men to enjoy intercourse once again.

"What is the measure of a man?" asks the poet. What is it that makes a man—and most important of all, makes him feel like a man? Throughout the ages, the first answer has always been: the ability to penetrate a woman's vagina with his erect penis, and to hold that erection long enough to ejaculate inside her. That made sense as long as the first purpose of sex was impregnation.

But even though procreation is now taking a back seat as a sex goal, the old definition is still powerful. So powerful in fact, that the man who cannot attain and hold an erection may lose all respect for himself as a man.

Within the last century, many causes for impotence have been discovered that were unthought of in earlier days. William Stekel, author of "Impotence in the Male", defines the condition as a "conflict between the brain and the spinal cord," and believes that all cases of impotence can be traced to emotional blocks—psychic inhibitions.

It is true that such may be the cause in the majority of cases—but not all. Impotence can often be the first symptom of a physical problem.

David became a victim of diabetes at the age of 42. His first indication was a spell of impotency; the diabetic condition was discovered when he consulted a doctor about his erection problem.

Prompt treatment brought David's diabetes under control medically and he found himself able to function sexually for several years. (In most cases, however, diabetic treatment does not restore a lost capacity for attaining erection). Then, suddenly impotency struck again. Two years of trials and failures to have sex with his wife led David to seek far-out remedies. He tried "cures" suggested at drugstore counters, and took hormone shots and pills prescribed by his doctor. Nothing worked.

David had always been a self-confident, jovial person. Now he gradually turned into a grouch, because he didn't feel like a man, and had a constant fear that he'd lose his wife, Vera. His desire for sex increased but penile erections remained impossible.

As time went on, a change came over the marriage. David and Vera gave up their double bed and got twin beds. They each started working overtime at their respective jobs, sometimes putting in 16 to 18 hours a day. They stopped touching each other. Without realizing it, they were avoiding each other.

Finally, Vera could no longer endure this sexless, unaffectionate life and urged her husband to consult the doctor about the damageing effect the impotency was having on their entire relationship.

Fortunately, by this time, David's physician had heard of a penile implant procedure being done in Des Moines by Dr. James Stallings. David had a penile implant six weeks after hearing the details.

One year after the operation, David feels that no one with his problem should be without a penile implant. He says he was going to pieces because he felt so ashamed of being impotent; knowing that he can function now has restored his old personality again.

He has intercourse from time to time, has no performance fears, and says sex is just as good as ever. His wife claims that, for her, sex is definitely better.

This couple was able to begin their new sex life four weeks after the surgery, and both know their marriage has been saved by the penile implant.

The penile implant technique consists of inserting two flexible silicone rubbers rods into the penis, in each corpus cavernosum (cave-like columns in the penis). The patient usually stays at the hospital three days; discomfort is kept at a minimum with ice packs and painkillers.

Contrary to misconceptions, this kind of implant does not give a man a perpetual erection, but provides enough firmness for penetration. David has to raise and lower his penis manually and can "tuck" it into jockey shorts or boxer trunks. He wears a regular bathing suit and says there's no noticeable bulge when wearing trousers. His sexual sensations are the same as before he became impotent; the implant hasn't taken anything from him except his affliction.

Like David most patients who have had a penile implant are satisfied with the results of the surgery. Dr. Robert A. Loeffler and Dr. Ronald E. Iverson, of Castro Valley, California, reported an 18-years experiencc with 250 penile implants in the Journal of Plastic & Reconstructive Surgery; all those followed up indicated they would have the procedure repeated for impotence in answer to that question.

Drs. Loeffler and Iverson found that the causes of impotence in their patients varied widely, but the most frequent receivers of implants were former cancer patients. Some of them had a rod implant inserted in the penis at the time of the cancer surgery, knowing they would not be able to obtain an erection afterward.

George S. is a typical cancer patient, suffering from carcinoma of the prostate gland. He had his testicles removed, as well as the prostate, and has since had X-ray and estrogen therapy. Both treatments can cause impotence. Even though George knows his cancer is spreading, he is concerned with the quality of his life at present, as is his doctor. He has, therefore, had both a penile implant and testicular implants. George feels that the ability to enjoy sex is vital to his well-being and justified the implants so he can feel like a whole man while he remains alive.

The second most frequent cause of impotence was psychic. All of those patients were evaluated by psychiatrists and given an implant to overcome long-term performance fears that resisted all efforts at counseling. Most doctors do not hesitate to do implants for psychic impotence after all other methods have been tried, without avail.

There is a long list of organic problems, which can cause impotence. Some are urology problems, some concern the nervous system. There are glandular problems, such as diabetes or hormonal imbalances. Vascular or vein problems, such as arteriosclerosis, probably pose the biggest difficulty in the older age group. In addition, various types of medicine are known to cause impotence; barbiturates, tranquilizers, and drugs used to control high blood pressure are among them. Alcohol and tobacco can also be a cause. Impotence from trauma has occurred in patients following fractures of the spine. One recipient of an implant sought help after exposure to weed killers had caused impotence.

Whatever the cause, long-term impotence can be relieved for the man who has a strong desire for sex and is capable of having an orgasm. The implant doesn't interfere with a normal erection or ejaculation.

There are, however, possible complications, which can arise after the operation. Infection or chronic pain, for instance, is sometimes experienced. Dead tissue may develop around the rods; all of the above complications may necessitate having the rods removed, which may leave the patient worse off than before having the operation done.

Dr. Harvey Lash of Palo Alto, California has been using an implant technique for over 15 years and stresses that this is not a panacea insofar as 100 percent solutions to impotency are concerned. He has tried a number of devices and keeps coming back to the simple rod.

He explains, "The ability to have intercourse or penetrate, as far as the mechanical part is concerned, depends on a lack of flexibility in the shaft of the penis. If pressure is applied to a limp penis, the shaft will buckle and intercourse is impossible. When a silicone rod is placed inside the corpus cavernosum (hollow bodies) of the penis, the shaft doesn't buckle."

Dr. Lash and his associates at the Palo Alto Medical Clinic operated at first only on patients who could not achieve an erection due to organic disease. Recently, however, they have placed implants in several psychologically impaired patients with gratifying results. In patients with premature ejaculation, intercourse can be continued after climax and ejaculation, even though the implant itself doesn't slow down the climax.

Doctors select candidates for the implant when they find that the implant when they find that the patient feels this aspect of his life is important enough to assume the risk of an operation and possible complications. There are few actual complications, but the operation is costly and is seldom covered totally by health insurance plans.

Doctor do thorough screening and testing on all prospective patients before they will perform the operation. Most patients who are accepted for the procedure are totally impotent—that is, they do not have even partial erections or ejaculations, mental health, too, is evaluated; some patients are considered too unstable, or psychotic, to have the operation.

Implants and surgical techniques vary as much as the reasons for having one. Dr. James Stallings feels that two rods give uniformly good results. He makes an incision in the pubic hair from the top, says that there is less risk of contamination with the incision there, and that the scar doesn't show. He places a flexible, silicone rubber rod (about 0.9 by 13.3 cm.) in each corpus cavernosum (hollow body), but picks the size (diameter and length) of the rods to suit the individual.

Dr. Harvey Lash feels two rods produce an undesirable position for the penis. He has experimented with an inflatable implant, a balloon-like device that simulates a normal erection's "hydraulic system."

Another inflatable implant was devised by Dr. Brantly Scott and two associates in Houston, Taxas; it is a reversible "pump." Silicone tubes are implanted in the penis, which are connected to a tiny hand-operated pump implanted inside the scrotum. An erection with this device increases the breadth of the penis, but may not increase the length. According to Dr. Lash, it has little, if any, advantage over the simple rod; and the fact that it involves a balloon, a reservoir, a pump, and several valves is overcomplicated and disconcerting. He is also has doubts about how long it will last.

A report in a recent issue of *New York Magazine* notes further complications: Sometimes the reservoir leaks, causing a return of impotency; sometimes the tubing can get tangled, causing a permanent erection.

So the single rod is Dr. Lash's preferred treatment, even though it does have some disadvantages. The rod does not have a fixed position, so a man must apply his hand firmly to his abdomen, almost as if he were holding a cigarette, in order to insert his penis into his partner's vagina. His movements then have to be rotary, rather than thrusting. Nonetheless, patients who have learned to use the device, after being totally impotent for a long time, are delighted to be able to have intercourse at all (whether their impotence is physical or psychological).

For many men, whose impotence springs from physical causes, penile implants have been a blessing. And in a number of large city hospitals, urologists are experimenting with different techniques. While psychological evaluation, as well as a full medical exploration, is recommended for all cases of impotence, a fairly simple operation can give new life to the man for whom all other solutions to his age-old problem have failed.

Chapter-25

Ageing and Sex

A large-scale survey of sex activities of ageing males has just been concluded. More than 800 men—ranging in age from 65 to well over 80—answered a series of question which had been sent to a list of persons who had distinguished themselves in various professional careers. *This total constitutes by far the largest number of men in this age group that has yet been studied.* The Kinsey study on the male, for example, reported having histories of only 87 white males and 39 Negro males past 60 years of age. Other studies have also involved a comparatively small number of males in this age group. This survey like the other preceding it, explodes many of the myths and false notions which most people still hold about the sexuality of people over 65. The most frequent idea one meets is the one that ageing is inevitably accompanied by sexual impotence. Closely associated with this notion is the concept that there is something shameful and "abnormal" about aged persons engageing in sexual activities. These two ideas are so widespread that aged persons themselves often believe them. Many older people are ashamed of their natural sex desires, and think there is something wrong with them when they have sex feelings. Quite often this sense of guilt has a bad psychological effect upon men. Expecting to be impotent, as they grow older, they actually become so as a result of their anticipation.

Only a handful of scientific studies of the sexual activities of the aged have been made. Scientific research in this field has been blocked by the traditional prejudice in our society not only against the idea of studying sexuality in general, but also particularly against studying the sex life of older people.

However, the few studies that have been made by physicians, psychologists, and sociologists all conclude universally that the sex drive remains strong in the sixth, seventh, eighth and even ninth decades of life, and that sexual impotence is not an inevitable biological consequence of growing old.

In order to add to the knowledge in this area, a survey was conducted. A committee for Geriatric Research was formed consisting of five medical doctors practicing in various fields. The committee addressed a questionnaire containing questions involving basic information about sexual activities to 6,000 men who were 65 years of age and over 832 rplies—representing 14% of the original 6,000—were received by the Committee. In order to ensure more careful and reliable responses, the six thousand persons were selected from lists of prominent persons who had achieved distinction in many professional fields. Among those responding, the largest groups consisted of educators, business leaders, attorneys, engineers, physicians, clergymen, and writers. The completed questionnaires contain a wealth of interesting information. A number of important enlightening facts are revealed by the responses which probably hold true for most aged men, particularly in the professional and middle classes.

Generally, the results of this study indicate that a majority of aged men not only are capable of natural satisfying sexual activities, but also actually at present do live healthy sex lives. The overwhelming majority of those who replied and completed the questionnaire were married. Specifically, 81% were married, 5% were widowed, 1% were single, and 13% were married but did not have an available partner with whom to engage in sexual activities. **Overall, the figures indicate that 70% of the married men surveyed 65 years of age and over engage regularly in sexual intercourse, and that the overwhelming majority of these have a satisfying sexual life with satisfactory sexual potency. Some general conclusion arrived at by examining the responses to the questionnaire are especially enlightening.**

Frequency of Coitus

The average frequency of coitus of the majority of the men was approximately four times a month. Obviously those with unsatisfactory potency have less frequent coitus than those with satisfactory powers. Yet a substantial group of even those with unsatisfactory sexual potency, namely 25% report engageing in sexual intercourse three or four times a month. It is interesting to note in the responses that lack of sexual desire is a strong element in discourageing more frequent coitus. This factor would seem to be related to the question of unhappiness in marriage and lack of arousal by one's partner as well as to the element of age. Where sexual impotence is a problem among married men, the sexual difficulty does not seem to be primarily related to any physical illness associated with ageing. For over 90% of all of the men reported that they did not have any physical disability, which could serve as a deterrent to more frequent coitus.

Sexual Potency

Most of the men who were impotent did not seek any medical treatment for this disability. This may have been because they automatically believed the false idea that impotence is an inevitable consequence of the ageing process. Since ageing itself could not be reversed, many undoubtedly felt that the impotence they experienced was also irreversible. This, of course, is a false notion, since many cases of impotence can be treated successfully at any age. Needless to say, such men have denied themselves unnecessarily many years of happy fulfilling sexual activities. A large number of the men who described themselves as impotent indicated that they had morning erections "occasionally" or "frequently." Although this is still an unsettled question medically, some physicians believe that this may indicate that there is no organic basis for impotence. This confirms the Kinsey investigation finding that morning erections usually persist for several years after a male has become completely impotent in other situations. No particular age was found to be an age at which men suddenly cease sex activity. Of 142 married men who described themselves as being impotent at the time of answering the questionnaire, fourteen said that sex activity had ceased between the ages of 40-59; fifty-three between the ages of 60-65; and seventy-five had ended their sex life at some time over the age of 65.

Fear of Heart Attack

It is important to note that the overwhelming majority answered that they were not deterred from coitus by fear of heart attack. Many doctors and scientists have often taken for granted that older people avoid sexual exertion because of this fear. This study shows that the sex drive is apparently much stronger than the fear of heart illness.

Masturbation

The objectivity and scientific validity of personal responses to questions about masturbation are often limited. The false notions and the deep guilts concerning masturbation with which most men and women grow up in our puritanical and repressive society are usually sufficient to supercharge responses concerning this practice with irrelevant notions and prejudices as well as a fear of answering truthfully. However, "yes" responses can generally be considered valid and true, while "no" answers cannot necessarily be trusted as factual. **Almost a quarter of the men answered that masturbation was a current practice. This was true of men with satisfactory potency, with unsatisfactory potency, and with total impotency. It should be noted, of course, that masturbation is more frequent among men of this social level at all ages.** It is usually accepted that people who have a satisfactory marital sex life engage in masturbation less often than people who have an unsatisfactory sex life. It is interesting to note that this notion is not confirmed by this study. For approximately the same percentage of the men who were impotent or reported unsatisfactory potency as the men with satisfactory potency currently engage in the practice of self-gratification.

This finding about masturbation in older men—all of whom had attained distinction in their professions—is perhaps the most startling finding in the survey. It certainly casts doubts upon beliefs held by some that masturbation is an immature and childish practice. The above represent a very few of the findings and possible conclusions which result from this special study of the sex life of men over 65 years of age. The most important finding is that a man in this age bracket can have, and many do have, perfectly happy, healthy, natural sexual desires and sexual experiences. Many of the problems of impotence in men over the age of 65 would seem to be caused by factors, which are similar to those causing impotence among younger men. Elimination of the general social bias which associates shame and guilt with sexual desires and sexual expression in older person would go a long way toward helping such individuals experience more fulfilling sex lives. **Certainly there seems to be no valid medical or scientific reason for aged people to believe that they are incapable to satisfactory sexual activities just because they are over 65 years age.**

Chapter-26

Fertility in Elderly Men

Puberty in boys and girls begins at 11 to 14 years of age with the production of cells: *spermatozoa* and *eggs*. Erection and ejaculation are the first signs of sexual maturity in boys.

In girls it is the appearance of the first menstrual bleeding (*menstruation*). The maturity of the eggs at this early age is usually not sufficient for fertilization. Full fertility develops a few years later.

In the woman, menstrual bleeding is an external sign of sexual and reproductive capacity. Between the ages of 45 and 50 the female sex glands cease their generative function, menstrual bleeding disappears, and the *climacteric* (change-of-life) occurs.

Is a man over sixty still potent and capable of reproducing? Is there in men, as in women, a definite age when generative function ceases? Do men of advanced years experience a condition resembling the *climacteric* of women?

The functional condition of the male reproductive glands may be determined either by microscopically studying the testicular tissue (*testicular biopsy*) or by examining the excretions of the sex glands (in the ejaculate or after prostate massage) for the presence of *spermatozoa*.

Research Findings

In clinical investigations, the contents of male sexual glands were expelled by rectal massage and examined microscopically for presence of spermatozoa. Rectal massage is a very simple and ordinary medical procedure, which may take place during an office visit. The expelled fluid was placed on slides and examined through a microscope. The finding was considered positive only when active living spermatozoa were seen in such a fresh preparation. With the living spermatozoa were also inactive dead spermatozoa.

These investigations involved 83 men from 60 to 92 years of age. Fifty-five of them showed living spermatozoa in the expelled fluid; spermatogenesis (production of spermatozoa) was still retained. In 36 of the 57 men over 70, reproductive-cell production was maintained. Five men between 80 and 92 years of age produced active spermatozoa.

The history of a patient, a 92-year-old man, is not atypical. This case showed a positive sperm finding four days before his death. His father died at the age of 84, and two of the father's *siblings* (brothers and sisters) died at 70 and 75 year of age. His mother died at 94, and her *siblings* died at 85 and 93. Two of the patient's five *siblings* died at 74 and 80, while there were still living at 85, 80, and 98 years of age. The patient had eight children: four of them died in their early ages; the other four were living at 50,54, 61, and 69 years of age.

Male change-of-life

We distinguish between two sexual capacities in man: *Potentia coeundi* and *Potentia generandi. Potentia coeundi* is the ability to perform the sex act; it depends up *erection ability and ejaculation. Potentia generandi* is ability to produce male sexual cells; it is *reproductive potency.*

Living spermatozoa in the secretion expelled from the genital organs of old men must not be regarded as unquestionable proof of their reproductive faculty. Such living spermatozoa do not necessarily indicate potency. They prove that the production of male sexual cells has not ceased in spite of age.

It is obvious that the production of the sexual cells in men may be maintained up to the most advanced age; it seems to be an extremely resistant vital process. There is no established age at which the functions of man's reproductive glands cease. If by change-of-life one means the discontinuance of the reproductive function of the genital glands, the climacteric does not occur in man.

In women, the change-of-life usually occurs between 45 and 50 years of age.

From the published observations, it is difficult to deduce very much regarding the sexual potency and reproductive capacity of the ageing man. It may probably be assumed that the preservation of spermatogenesis to a most advanced age is influenced by hormones. But we do not know which hormone processes are instrumental in the organism of the ageing man. According to our present knowledge, the testicles possess a twofold inner secretory function. One of these is related to *spermatogenesis,* but in a manner not yet fully understood.

No change-of-life occurs in the human male. The decrease in sexual activity is a result of general wear and tear of the male organism with advancing age. This becomes adversely affected through psychological factors when the man, in spite of decreased sexual ability, has the desire to engage in sexual activity and is not in a condition to do so. Beacuse of psychological depression, his poteney may be still further decreased. A vicious cycle may occur when the man does not realize that it is more expedient to let nature run her course undisturbed, instead of pursuing her in vain.

Chapter-27

Contraception

Reproduction involves a woman's egg being Fertilized by a man's sperm, which is called Conception. Here we explore the ways of preventing Conception: *contraception*.

The most statistically perfect method of contraception is abstinence, which is defined as 'denial of the appetites"—in this case, sexual appetite. Abstinence is not a realistic method of contraception for most adults. Contraceptive potions and devices are mentioned in historical records from thousands of years ago—interest in and use of contraception did not begin with the Pill, the diaphragm, or the condom.

Even though we now have several effective methods of contraception, modern couples often don't have a much clearer idea of how to have sex and not become pregnant than did the Egyptians or other ancient cultures.

Although the presence of sperm in semen was not discovered until 1677, we know that most civilizations understood the connection between pregnancy and intercourse. Since ancient times, people have attempted to neutralize the fertilizing effects of intercourse.

An Egyptian papyrus from 1850 B.C. lists such contraceptive methods as crocodile dung mixed with a paste to form a pessary (a substance or device placed in the vagina to prevent sperm from entering the uterus). The effectiveness of this method was not reported, but based on what we now know about hygiene, putting dung in the vagina is clearly not a good idea. A 1550 B.C. papyrus describes a tamponlike pessary made from lint and then coated with ground acacia (a type of tree), colocynth (a fruit-bearing plant), dates, and honey. This advice might have been somewhat effective, because acacia breaks down into lactic acid, an ingredient in modern spermicides. Records from Greek, Roman, Islamic, Persian, and other ancient cultures all include recipes for potions to be swallowed or inserted into the body to prevent pregnancy.

The Bible, the Talmud, and writings from other religions also mention various methods, including coitus interruptus (withdrawal), the use of vaginal sponges, and the preparation of contraceptive concoctions. According to some historians, the biblical story of Onan in the book of Genesis (33:9) verifies that those ancient peoples understood the connection between intercourse and pregnancy; it serves as one illustration that they knew about coitus interruptus at the time.

The first description of a condom appeared in 1564. Made of linen, it was initially promoted as a protection against syphilis (it didn't work). In the 1700s condoms began to be made from animal intestines and were widely used for contraception. By that time, shops specializing in contraceptive products had appeared in Europe.

The history of contraception in the United States began in the mid-1700s with the importing of Hooper's Female Pills from England. A principal ingredient in the pill was aloes, an abortifacient (a drug that induces miscarriage).

Publications dating from 1830 recommended coitus interruptus, vaginal sponges, condoms, and douching (which doesn't work) to prevent pregnancy. Charles Goodyear discovered how to vulcanize rubber in 1843, and shortly thereafter rubber condoms were manufactured in large numbers. By 1880, one author noted that "probably more than one half of the adult population in the U.S is resorting to birth control".

Around 1880, the diaphragm was invented in Germany, followed in 1909 by an intrauterine device (IUD). The idea that there is a "safe" time in a woman's cycle to have sex also become popular in the nineteenth century. Unfortunately, abstinence from sex was recommended from the time of menstrual bleeding until *midcylce*—a schedule that makes conception *more,* not *less,* likely. Not until the 1930s did researchers in Japan and Austria discover that women release an egg at midcycle—not immediately after menstruation, as had been believed.

Until the Food and Drug Administration approved the first birth control pill in 1960, the diaphragm used with spermicidal jellies was the method recommended most frequently by physicians and women's clinics in the United States.

CONTRACEPTIVE METHODS

Every person—or, preferably, each couple through mutual discussion—should choose a contraceptive method based on accurate information about failure rates, reversibility (for the time when they do decide to start a family), safety, and their personal health status.

Age, life style, and personal values also play an important role in choosing a contraceptive method. We now also know that a person's health and later fertility can be affected by sexually transmitted disease (STDs) such as chlamydia and that viruses that cause genital warts and AIDS. Therefore, people must also consider those methods, which offer effective protection against STDs. It is also true that the "best" choice for contraception at one point in a person's life may not be the "best" at another time—as general health, circumstances, or relationships change.

There are three basic concepts to keep in mind as you evaluate various contraceptive methods: Not using any method for one year (leaving it to chance) will result in pregnancy for 90 out of 100 couples; no contraceptive method is 100 percent effective; and the risk of dying from any approved contraceptive method is far smaller than the risk of dying from pregnancy and childbirth for the vast majority of women.

This chapter is devoted to some specific contraceptive methods, arranged from the most to the least effective when used consistently and according to instructions.

1. VASECTOMY AND 2. TUBAL STERILIZATION

Surgical sterilization, whether vasectomy for men or tubal sterilization for women, is considered the most effective form of contraception available to date. It is also the most popular among married couples age 30 and older.

Vasectomy means cutting a man's vas deferens the two tubes the carry sperm from where they are produced in each testicle up into his body on their journey toward the penis. These tubes can be easily reached through a small opening made in the scrotum. The result is that no sperm can reach

the area inside the body where semen is pooled for ejaculation.

Tubal ligation literally means, "tying" a woman's Fallopian tubes, the two tubes through which eggs from the ovaries travel to the uterus and inside which sperm meet the egg for fertilization. There are different ways of performing a tubal sterilization, all of which involve surgery to go inside a woman's body (either through the abdomen or vagina) to cut, burn, tie, clip, or otherwise block the tubes.

The failure rate (when pregnancy occurs, or when sperm still appear in the ejaculate) following vasectomy is 160 for every 100,000 men on a lifetime basis. Lifetime failure rates following tubal sterilization vary from 276 to 326 per 100,000 women, depending on the specific surgical technique used. If pregnancy does occur women who have had a tubal ligation have a higher risk of ectopic pregnancy (when a fertilized egg implants in the tube rather than in the uterus), a life-threatening situation.

Clearly, vasectomy for the man is a more effective and far safer choice for a couple than is tubal sterilization for the woman. It is also less expensive and carries a lower risk of complications following the procedure.

Unfortunately, there are widespread myths that vasectomy reduces a man's sex drive, makes him unable to ejaculate, or carries long-term health risks—none of which are true.

Both vasectomy and tubal sterilization must be considered permanent and irreversible, despite claims to the contrary. Another disadvantage is that neither procedure provides protection against STDs; some researchers, however, speculate that in the case of those STDs carried by sperm, vasectomy may reduce risks for a man's sexual partner.

3 ORAL HORMONAL CONTRACEPTIVES (THE PILL)

The next most effective method of contraception after sterilization is taking oral hormonal pills (the Pill), containing a combination of an estrogen and a *progestin* or *a progestin* alone. The failure rate is 2 to 3 women out of every 100 women who take them for one year.

One risk of using a progestin-only pill is that if pregnancy results, there is a greater chance of ectopic (tubal) pregnancy.

The Pill works by tricking the body into altering the amounts and the pattern of natural hormones released by the ovaries. The result is that eggs are not usually released, the cervical mucus remains impenetrable to sperm, and the uterine lining does not permit implantation of a zygote even if an egg and sperm were to meet. The reduced build-up of the lining of the uterus is also why many women have lighter menstrual flow while they take the Pill.

Some women should not take the Pill. These include women with previous blood clots, those who have suffered a stroke, coronary artery disease, or breast cancer—and women who smoke. Others who may be at increased risk of serious side effects are women with high blood pressure, diabetes, gall bladder disease, or irregular menstrual cycles.

Every women taking the Pill should memorize the following danger signals and report them to her physician or clinic immediately: severe abdominal pain, severe chest pain, or shortness of breath; severe headache, dizziness, weakness, of numbness; loss or blurring of vision; speech problems; or severe pain in the calf or thigh. If women taking the Pill reported these warning signs promptly, their physicians could carefully evaluate the cause and can stop the pill immediately.

Other health benefits of taking the Pill for some women include reduced menstrual cramps, lower incidence of ovarian cysts, reduced PMS symptoms, more regular cycles, and decreased incidence of fibrocystic breast problems. The Pill seems to have a dramatic effect in lowering the risk of PID (pelvic inflammatory disease). Studies in Europe and the United States report a 50 to 70 percent reduction in hospitalization for PID if a woman is taking the Pill, particularly if she has taken it for more than twelve months.

Another beneficial reason for choosing the Pill is that it is highly reversible. When a woman decides to get pregnant, all she need do is switch to a barrier method for at least one full cycle. This enables her body to resume its natural hormonal cycling; then she stops using any form of contraception.

One of the drawbacks of choosing the Pill for contraception is that it does not provide protection against STDs. The Pill may also reduce the effectiveness of antibiotics used to treat

STDs. The Pill may also reduce the effectiveness of antibiotics used to treat STDs—and taking antibiotics for any infection can also reduce the effectiveness of the Pill.

4 INTRAUTERINE DEVICE (IUD)

An IUD is a device inserted into the uterus and left there to prevent conception. Legend has it that the first IUD was used in Arabia, where camel drivers put stones into their camels' uteri before leaving on long journeys so they would not become pregnant during the trip. Over the centuries hundreds of such devices have been tried with various materials (silver, gold, copper, and plastic) and shapes (loops, spirals, Ts, and 7s). It appears that IUDs work by chemically altering the uterine environment thus interfering with the sperm as they travel through the uterus, before they meet the egg.

Only two types of IUDs are currently available: Paraguard (a copper-bearing device) and *Progestasert* (a progestin-releasing device).

Because IUDs must be removed on a regular basis (for example, Copper-7s and Copper-Ts are to be removed three years after insertion), many women must now decide which of the two available types of IUDs to use—or change to a different method of contraception.

The failure rate of the Progestasert for 100 women using it for one year is 2.6 for women who have not had a previous pregnancy and 1.8 for women who have.

Paraguard has been in use for a little over one year, so not much data are available, but its failure rate appears to be low (0.5 percent—5 out of 1000). It can be left in place for four years—an advantage because the highest rate of infection with IUDs occurs in the first few months after insertion. This is thought to be because the IUD has the opportunity to pick up infectious organisms from the vagina or cervix during insertion.

Currently most clinics suggest certain women should not use an IUD due to the somewhat increased risk of PID (Pelvic Inflammatory Disease), a condition that can reduce fertility by causing scarring of the Fallopian tubes. Women are at higher risk of developing PID if they are not in a sexual relationship that is mutually exclusive; they are at high risk for catching STDs or have symptoms of an STD; or they have a history of ectopic (tubal) pregnancy.

It is recommended that women in low-risk groups who do decide to use an IUD have it inserted by a physician or at a clinic experienced in doing the procedure.

So far we have explored contraceptive methods that work by disrupting the travel of sperm through the male reproductive tract (vasectomy), disrupting the travel of eggs and sperm through the female reproductive tract (tubal sterilization), reducing the release of eggs (the Pill), or interfering with the travel of sperm (IUD).

Barrier methods work differently. In these methods, sperm are trapped at the point of ejaculation (condoms), retained in the vagina so they cannot swim through the woman's cervix (diaphragms, sponges, and cervical caps), or inactivated with a chemical (spermicides—foams, creams, jellies, and suppositories).

Another major difference between barrier methods and those discussed earlier is that the use of barrier methods is directly linked to the time intercourse occurs and therefore involves conscious planning and preparation. You have to acknowledge that intercourse may occur and have the condom or other barrier device ready for use.

Barrier methods must also be used each and every time intercourse occurs. Used consistently and correctly, some barrier methods can have failure rates nearly as low as the Pill. In addition, they can provide good protection against many STDs and are highly reversible. When a couple desires a pregnancy they simply stop using the method. With exception of the diaphragm and cervical cap, which must be properly fitted and therefore prescribed by a health clinic or physician, barrier devices do not require a prescription, are widely available. Negative side effects or health risks with barrier methods are very rare; very few people report allergic reactions to spermicides or latex rubber.

In fact, barrier methods, especially when used in combinations (such as condoms or diaphragms with spermicides that have nonoxynol-9 or octoxynol as an ingredient) can provide one of the safest and most effective methods of contraception available if used correctly and used each time.

NOTE:

Oil or petroleum-based lubricants destroy latex rubber condoms, diaphragms, and cervical caps. You may not be able to see the damage but microscopic hoes through which sperm and infectious organisms can escape are likely to occur. Within 60 seconds, holes appear which are big enough for some STD organisms to pass through, and soon after these devices deteriorate enough for sperm to get through. Therefore, products like Vaseline, baby oil, Crisco, butter, Nivea, Vaseline Intensive Care, or other lotions should not be used with these contraceptive methods. When more vaginal lubrication is desired, use only water-based products like K-Y jelly or *Lubrin* inserts.

5 CONDOMS

A condom is a sheath made of latex rubber or animal intestine (sometimes called "skins") that is rolled onto an erect penis. Only latex condoms have been shown to protect against the smaller-size STD viruses such as HIV (the AIDS virus) and hepatitis-B. Latex condoms come in various sizes, shapes, thickness, colors, and textures and are widely available.

6 DIAPHRAGMS

A diaphragm is a flexible metal ring covered by a dome-shaped piece of latex rubber. A tablespoon of spermicidal cream or jelly is placed inside the dome and then spread into a thin film around the rim. The diaphragm is then placed high inside the woman's vagina, covering and completely surrounding her cervix. It must be inserted shortly before intercourse (spermicidal gradually loses effectiveness) and must remain in place for six hours after intercourse. If a second intercourse occurs before the six hours are up, place more *spermicide* into the vagina without removing the diaphragm. A diaphragm must be fitted and prescribed by a physician or health clinic, lasts about two years with proper care.

7 CERVICAL CAP

A cervical cap is small latex, thimble-shaped version of a diaphragm that fits over only the cervix (rather than against the vaginal walls like a diaphragm). It must be fitted and prescribed by a physician or clinic. It, too, is used with a spermicide that is placed inside the cap. It is inserted shortly before intercourse and must be kept in place for six hours after having intercourse. Caps should be cleaned and stored like diaphragms, checked for wear, and replaced every twelve to eighteen months.

8 SPERMICIDES

Spermicides are available in various forms: foam, creams, jellies, dissolvable tablets, and suppositories. Spermicides do not require a prescription, but directions for use must be carefully followed.

Used correctly, spermicides work in two ways. The active chemical in a spermicide literally disables sperm, and the base—the foam, cream, or jelly—covers the cervix, acting as a mechanical barrier. An important additional advantage is that if the spermicides contains nonoxynol-9 or octoxynol, it also apparently provides protection against many STDs: Nisseria gonorrhoeae (gonorrhea), trichomonas vaginalis, herpes virus, AIDS virus, Treponema *pallidum, Ureaplasma urealycticum,* and perhaps chlamydia.

Creams, jellies, and foams should be used according to instructions on the container and begin to lose effectiveness after thirty minutes. Tablets and suppositories require ten to fifteen minutes to dissolve before they become protective. All should be inserted high in the vagina, as close as possible to the cervical opening. Foam appears to provide the best covering of the cervix, tablets and suppositories the least. Used alone, spermicides have a typical failure rate of about 18 to 21 per 100 women per year. They are more effective when used with another form of contraception, such as a diaphragm or condom.

Spermicides are widely available, do not require a prescription, are relatively inexpensive, and generally considered safe.

9 CONTRACEPTIVE SPONGE

This is a small, round polyurethane sponge with one dimpled side that fits at the end of the vagina over the cervix. The other side has a loop for removal. Each soft sponge has a spermicide that is activated by moistening it in water before insertion. It must be left in place for eight hours after having sex, then removed and discarded. If you have sex again before it's time to remove the sponge, add an application of spermicide into the vagina without removing the sponge. The failure rate for the contraceptive sponge is around 18 percent (10 to 20 of 100 women per year).

10 WITHDRAWAL (COITUS INTERRUPTUS)

With a failure of 23 percent, withdrawal is clearly not considered one of the more effective methods of contraception. However, for those with strong religious convictions, it remains one of the few options that has at least some effect.

Your husband doesn't have to actually ejaculate inside of you in order for you to become pregnant. Sperm have been found in the clear pre-ejaculatory fluid, which can appear at the tip of the penis during arousal long before ejaculation occurs.

You can also become pregnant if your husband withdraws after he has begun to ejaculate. There are more sperm in the first one or two spurts than in the later ejaculatory spasms; and sometimes the male isn't able to withdraw until ejaculation has already begun.

You can also become pregnant if your partner withdraws, then ejaculates near, though not inside, the vaginal opening (on the labia or other parts of the vulva). Sperms are strong swimmers (faster for their size than the greatest Olympic champions) and can swim relatively long distances and around many obstacles to reach their goal.

Withdrawal doesn't physically harm either one of you, but it can pose other problems. It can affect the natural sequence of intercourse if both partners are only thinking "Will he stop in time?" there is the chance that withdrawal can lead to sexual difficulties because both partners are focusing on only this one aspect of the male sexual response. Suddenly stopping intercourse can leave the woman dissatisfied unless other means are used for her to achieve orgasm, either before or after intercourse.

Some researchers have stressed that failure rates for coitus interruptus can be lower for those men who are aware of and can control their point of ejaculatory inevitability.

Unfortunately, younger men who attempt this method have rarely gained this kind of control because their experience is limited to masturbation, which is often done quickly. But couples, who care for each other, help each other enjoy sex and orgasms, and know each other well enough to help the man gain control many do better than the statistics imply. Although far from perfect, this method is better than using nothing at all.

11 FERTILITY AWARENESS METHODS

A woman's egg is only available for fertilization for a day or less in each cycle, but sperm can reach the egg from semen deposited in the vagina anytime from approximately eight days before ovulation plus the day of ovulation.

The goal of fertility awareness (also called "natural family planning" or the "rhythm method") is to predict when ovulation will occur in a given cycle so that a couple who does not want to conceive does not have sex anytime near the woman's fertile time.

The basic varieties of fertility awareness are the calendar, basal body temperature, and cervical mucus methods. The typical failure rate for fertility awareness methods is high—24 pregnancies out of 100 couples who use the method for one year. To achieve a better rate couples must have good training; both partners must be committed to abstaining from intercourse during the entire fertile time; multiple fertility awareness methods should be used; and instructions must be closely followed every day. When all this is done and the woman also has fairly regular cycles, the failure rate can sometimes be reduced to around 2 to 10 pregnancies per 100 couples.

The CALENDAR method is based on the assumption that ovulation will occur about fourteen days before the next menstrual flow begins. Ovulation occurs at approximately the middle of a reproductive cycle, which begins with the first day of menstrual flow of one period and ends on the first day of flow in the next. A woman keeps records of her first day of menstrual flow for six full cycles (not all cycles will last the same number of days). She identifies the shortest cycle, takes that number of days, and subtracts 18—this is considered the first "unsafe" day after each menstrual flow begins. She then identifies her longest cycle, takes that number of days, and subtracts 11—this is thought to be her last "unsafe" day in a cycle.

Then the couple does not have intercourse on any "unsafe" days. For most couples, this means no intercourse for at least ten consecutive days in the middle of every cycle. This method, however, does not take into account the fact that many women have such irregular cycles that future "unsafe" days cannot be accurately predicted from records of past cycles.

The basal body temperature (BBT)—basal means "resting"—method helps some couples because it can show when ovulation has actually occurred in a cycle. In many women basal temperature rises by 0.4 to 0.8 degree Fahrenheit within twenty-four hours after ovulation and stays higher until her next menstrual flow. This rise is due to an increase in progesterone produced by the corpus luteum. Using a special thermometer (one that shows a range only from 96°F to 100°F, making it easier to see fractions of degree) a woman takes her basal temperature each morning before she gets out of bed, drinks or eats anything, or smokes. Then she records the temperature on a chart. After keeping such charts for six months, the couple should theoretically be able to see the day ovulation occurred in past cycles. To prevent pregnancy, no intercourse is permitted for at least seven days before the temperature is expected to rise in future cycles, plus the three days after it actually has risen in each cycle.

Although slightly better than the calendar method, the BBT failure is still around 20 per 100 couples per year, except for those couples who follows the so-called "strict" BBT method; no intercourse is permitted from the first day of menstrual flow until four days after the BBT has risen. Having sex only on those few remaining days (for many couples this would mean only ten or eleven days in each cycle) does yield a lower failure rate—6 pregnancies per 100 couples per year.

A third awareness technique—checking for the consistency of cervical mucus—is also recommended by some groups. This method is based on the theory that the estrogen level peaks just before ovulation. As a women's level of estrogen rises in the first part of her cycle it not only stimulates growth of an egg but also affects her cervix, producing more mucus and of a different type. The color and texture differ from cervical mucus at other stages of the cycle. At the highest estrogen levels the mucus looks like raw egg white, can be slowly stretched between the fingertips to a strand the length of four inches, and makes a woman feel wet, slippery, or oily around the vaginal opening. At other times, the woman's vulval area feels drier, the mucus looks more yellow or milky and will not stretch between the fingertips.

Although most women using the mucus method monitor their cervical mucus at the vaginal opening, some use a speculum (the instrument used by a gynecologist to open the vagina so the cervix can be seen) and a mirror to look at the cervix itself. These women can also look for changes in the os (the opening in the cervix). The os is closed during most of *the cycle, but begins to open around the same time that mucus production increases. This permits sperm to enter more easily around the time of ovulation. The cervix also opens at menstruation.*

As with other awareness methods, mucus observations are recorded on a chart, and a couple wishing to avoid pregnancy has intercourse only on those days after ovulation is over in one cycle up the first day of menstrual flow in the next cycle. Then they may also have intercourse on alternate days after menstrual flow stops, so long as the "egg white" type of mucus has not appeared. In one study of couples using only the mucus method, the failure rate was nearly 40 per 100 couples.

The major problem with all these fertility awareness methods is that many women do not have temperature changes or mucus changes that match the patterns these methods are based on. Also, a wide array of common events can change temperature (having a cold or the flu, sleeping late, stress) or change mucus secretions (vaginal infections, taking medications, being sexually aroused) for even those women who are usually regular and who are conscientious about monitoring and recording observations.

All of the fertility awareness methods are highly reversible when a couple decides to start a family and most cost nothing or are inexpensive, but none offer any protection against STDs.

Other Books by Same Author:

- Encyclopedia of Medicine and Surgery
- Sexual Debility and it's Treatment
- A book of Gynaecology and Obstetrics
- Injection Therapy
- Modern Diagnosis and Treatment
- Male Sexual Disorders and Their Treatment
- Overcoming sexual disorders and Sexually Tansmitted Diseases

Books Translated by Same Author:

- Medical Instruments
- First Aid
- Food and Nutrition
- Churchill Livingstone's: Pocket Medical Dictionary
- Handbook of Preventive and Social Medicine

12 DOUCHING

Douching is forcing a liquid into the vagina and letting it drain back out. The failure rate for douching is 40 percent (out of 100 women using this method for one year, 40 will become pregnant). Moreover, most douching liquids offer no protection against STDs, as do some other methods of contraception, and new data have revealed that douching may increase the risk of developing PID and its consequences—infertility and ectopic pregnancy.

NOTE:

Except for sexual abstinence, none of the various contraceptive surgeries, products, devices, and other methods currently available *are* 100 percent effective. Statistically, even among the most conscientious, careful couples using the most effective methods in exactly the prescribed way, a few will experience a contraceptive failure.